VOLUME FIFTY TWO

INTERNATIONAL REVIEW OF RESEARCH IN DEVELOPMENTAL DISABILITIES

Identifying and Addressing the Social Issues Experienced by Individuals with IDD

VOLUME FIFTY TWO

INTERNATIONAL REVIEW OF RESEARCH IN DEVELOPMENTAL DISABILITIES

Identifying and Addressing the Social Issues Experienced by Individuals with IDD

Edited by

MARISA H. FISHER
Dept. of Counseling, Educational Psychology, & Special Education
Michigan State University
East Lansing, MI
United States

ELSEVIER

ACADEMIC PRESS
An imprint of Elsevier

Academic Press is an imprint of Elsevier
50 Hampshire Street, 5th Floor, Cambridge, MA 02139, United States
525 B Street, Suite 1800, San Diego, CA 92101-4495, United States
125 London Wall, London EC2Y 5AS, United Kingdom
The Boulevard, Langford Lane, Kidlington, Oxford OX5 1GB, United Kingdom

First edition 2017

ISBN: 978-0-12-811822-1
ISSN: 2211-6095

For information on all Academic Press publications visit our website at https://www.elsevier.com/books-and-journals

Publisher: Zoe Kruze
Acquisition Editor: Kirsten Shankland
Editorial Project Manager: Charlotte Rowley
Production Project Manager: James Selvam
Designer: Mark Rogers

Typeset by TNQ Books and Journals

CONTENTS

CONTRIBUTORS

Ryan Adams
Cincinnati Children's Hospital Medical Center, Cincinnati, OH, United States

Somer Bishop
University of California–San Francisco, San Francisco, CA, United States

Erik W. Carter
Vanderbilt University, Nashville, TN, United States

Michael J. Cull
Tennessee Department of Children's Services, Nashville, TN, United States

Leopold M.G. Curfs
Maastricht University, Maastricht, The Netherlands;
The Governor Kremers Centre, Maastricht, The Netherlands

Richard A. Epstein
Chapin Hall Center for Children at the University of Chicago, Chicago, IL, United States

Mary Hanley
Durham University, Durham, United Kingdom

Brooke Ingersoll
Michigan State University, East Lansing, MI, United States

Connie Kasari
University of California Los Angeles, Los Angeles, CA, United States

Gerjo Kok
Maastricht University, Maastricht, The Netherlands;
The Governor Kremers Centre, Maastricht, The Netherlands

Emma Lough
Durham University, Durham, United Kingdom;
Newcastle University, Newcastle upon Tyne, United Kingdom

Joshua B. Plavnick
Michigan State University, East Lansing, MI, United States

Deborah M. Riby
Durham University, Durham, United Kingdom

Ellen Ridley
Durham University, Durham, United Kingdom

Dilana Schaafsma
Maastricht University, Maastricht, The Netherlands;
Fontys University of Applied Sciences, Eindhoven, The Netherlands;
The Governor Kremers Centre, Maastricht, The Netherlands

Stephanie Shire
University of California Los Angeles, Los Angeles, CA, United States

Kyle Sterrett
University of California Los Angeles, Los Angeles, CA, United States

Joke M.T. Stoffelen
Maastricht University, Maastricht, The Netherlands;
Zorgbelang Gelderland-Utrecht, Arnhem, The Netherlands;
The Governor Kremers Centre, Maastricht, The Netherlands

Julie Lounds Taylor
Vanderbilt University Medical Center, Nashville, TN, United States

Richard C. Urbano
Vanderbilt Kennedy Center, Nashville, TN, United States;
Vanderbilt University Medical Center, Nashville, TN, United States

Alison Vehorn
Vanderbilt Kennedy Center, Nashville, TN, United States

Zachary Warren
Vanderbilt Kennedy Center, Nashville, TN, United States;
Vanderbilt University Medical Center, Nashville, TN, United States;
Vanderbilt University, Nashville, TN, United States

PREFACE

Although the social difficulties of individuals with intellectual and developmental disabilities (IDD) vary based on several factors—including age, gender, and specific diagnosis—most individuals with IDD experience social problems beyond those of individuals without disabilities. Such social issues can take the form of trouble developing and maintaining friendships; interacting or conversing with others; understanding social cues and social nuances; and engaging in romantic relationships. These social difficulties can have secondary effects, as they can impact the parent–child bond, the educational experience, the ability to obtain and maintain employment, and even the ability to live independently.

Further, social difficulties are sometimes linked to experiences with victimization. As children, individuals with IDD are at increased risk of experiencing abuse at the hands of their parents and other caregivers. As they enter the school years, individuals with IDD are, compared to typically developing age-mates, more likely to experience bullying and other forms of peer victimization. And, as adults, individuals with IDD are at increased risk of being exploited (e.g., financially) and of experiencing physical and sexual abuse.

Given the high risk of a lifetime of victimization, it is critical to understand and address the social issues experienced by individuals with IDD. If such concerns can be addressed early, it may be possible to prevent the exposure to negative social experiences later. This special issue of *International Review of Research in Developmental Disabilities* contains chapters addressing both the prevalence and risk factors for social issues and victimization of people with IDD across the life span and presents important approaches to interventions to help address these problems.

Risk for victimization begins in early childhood, as children with IDD (compared to those without disabilities) are at increased risk of experiencing child abuse. Given their particular social and communication impairments, children with autism spectrum disorder (ASD) may be at increased risk for child abuse. Previous research findings, however, conflict about the prevalence of child abuse, with some studies indicating that children with ASD are not more likely to experience child abuse. In their chapter, Richard Urbano, Richard Epstein, Michael Cull, Alison Vehorn, and Zachary Warren first describe the methodological limitations in previous research, before presenting a new approach for determining the prevalence of maltreatment among children with ASD. Specifically, the authors describe how the Autism and Developmental Disabilities Monitoring Network database can be linked to data from Child Protective Services to identify those children with ASD who have been referred for child abuse investigations. The authors conclude by presenting preliminary findings of the database they created to identify the prevalence of child abuse among children with ASD.

In addition to the risk of abuse at the hands of the parent, young children with IDD also experience social difficulties that impact their ability to form and maintain friendships. Again, the social and communication impairments experienced by children with ASD make these children particularly vulnerable to friendship troubles. Intervention programs designed to teach social and friendship skills to preschool and elementary school age children could help to address friendship difficulties and change the negative trajectory for youth with ASD. To this end, Kyle Sterrett, Stephanie Shire, and Connie Kasari conducted a systematic review of this research to describe and examine the effectiveness of interventions designed to target the development of friendships, peer networks, and discrete social skills in young children with ASD. Given the importance of this information, the authors identify the need for additional research for evidence-based interventions for children with ASD.

As individuals with IDD and ASD reach adolescence, social problems continue to be a barrier to the formation of friendships and subsequently increase risk for peer victimization. In Chapter 3, Ryan Adams, Somer Bishop, and Julie Lounds Taylor present the research related to negative peer experiences in adolescents with ASD. These authors not only describe what is known about peer victimization toward individuals with ASD but they also identify several methodological limitations inherent in past ASD peer victimization research. Through a unique comparison of individuals with ASD to those who are obese, the authors end their chapter by providing preliminary evidence of the impact of peer victimization on the mental health outcomes of adolescents with ASD. These data are used to support the call for further research and the need to develop interventions that address the unique social challenges of individuals with IDD (including ASD). The authors argue that interventions should not only target individuals with ASD (e.g., in interventions targeting social deficits) but should also aim to change peer attitudes toward individuals with IDD/ASD.

Following up on this suggestion, the next two chapters present research on both of these approaches. Joshua Plavnick and Brooke Ingersoll address the need for social skills training for adolescents with ASD, through the development of a video-based group social skills instruction program. The authors first describe the iterative development process of the program and how the program was informed by the implementation science approach and by recent recommendations for ASD intervention developers. The end result was a promising video-based group social skills instruction program designed in collaboration with public school professionals and implemented in a community setting (e.g., the public high school). The authors end their chapter by presenting outcomes for 17 adolescents with ASD who participated in the social skills training.

Parallel to the need to work directly with individuals with ASD and IDD, Erik Carter presents peer support arrangements as an evidence-based approach for supporting students with intellectual disabilities in inclusive educational settings. Carter provides evidence for the effectiveness of peer supports and how they can not only address the social concerns of individuals with IDD, but they can also help support the academic success and inclusive education for students with IDD. He reviews the research, describing how this intervention approach has evolved to support students with varying needs, and he describes the components for effective implementation.

Although most of this volume's chapters are specific to individuals with ASD, individuals with other forms of IDD also experience social problems that must be addressed. Individuals with Williams syndrome present with a unique behavioral profile that includes hypersocial behavior and a tendency to approach and engage strangers. Although such friendly behaviors can be considered cute and endearing in early childhood, these same behaviors can increase the risk for social victimization in the adolescent and adult years. Raising awareness to this concern, Deborah Riby, Ellen Ridley, Emma Lough, and Mary Hanley provide an overview of the social issues experienced by individuals with Williams syndrome, before explaining how these individuals can be taken advantage of, both in the real world and online. Riby and colleagues then present a case study of an interview with a young woman with Williams syndrome and her mother. Through qualitative analysis, the authors provide a real-world example of how the social behavior of this woman with Williams syndrome presents the very real risk of victimization. The authors end with a call for intervention research to address the social vulnerability of individuals with Williams syndrome.

Finally, Joke Stoffelen, Dilana Schaafsma, Gerjo Kok, and Leopold Curfs address the incredibly important, yet seldom discussed topic of sexuality and sexual health for individuals with IDD. Stoffelen and colleagues give a broad overview of the sexual difficulties experienced by individuals with IDD and the need for additional research to understand the sexual needs of individuals with IDD. The authors provide information on ways their colleagues in the Netherlands are able to support the sexual health of individuals with IDD. Their review highlights the importance of expanding such research and intervention into other countries.

Overall, then, the chapters within IRRDD's Volume 52 focus on identifying and addressing the social issues experienced by individuals with IDD (and most specifically, ASD). The chapters not only present important data about the lifetime risk for victimization, but they also provide important approaches to intervention. Through these reviews it becomes clear that more work must be done to support individuals with IDD/ASD and to decrease their risk of social victimization. I hope these chapters are able to provide the impetus for future research in such a critical area. It was an honor to be invited to serve as a guest editor for this special issue of IRRDD. I thank each contributor for making this edition a priority, along with all of the other priorities they face every day. I also thank the reviewers for providing helpful and insightful reviews to the authors. I thank Dr. Robert Hodapp and Dr. Debbie Fidler for inviting me and trusting me to take on the job of guest editor. Finally, thank you to Charlotte Rowley at Elsevier for her patience and for keeping me on track with this special issue of IRRDD.

Marisa H. Fisher
July 27, 2017

CHAPTER ONE

Autism and Child Maltreatment: A Population-Based, Record Linkage Methodology for Studying Children Referred to Child Protective Services

Richard C. Urbano[*,§,1], **Richard A. Epstein**[¶], **Michael J. Cull**[||], **Alison Vehorn**[*], **Zachary Warren**[*,§,#]

[*]Vanderbilt Kennedy Center, Nashville, TN, United States
[§]Vanderbilt University Medical Center, Nashville, TN, United States
[¶]Chapin Hall Center for Children at the University of Chicago, Chicago, IL, United States
[||]Tennessee Department of Children's Services, Nashville, TN, United States
[#]Vanderbilt University, Nashville, TN, United States
[1]Corresponding author: E-mail: richard.urbano@gmail.com

Contents

International Review of Research in Developmental Disabilities, Volume 52
ISSN 2211-6095
http://dx.doi.org/10.1016/bs.irrdd.2017.07.005

Abstract

In this article, we demonstrate the use of linked, population-level data to examine how children with autism spectrum disorder (ASD) are processed by a state protective services agency. Although there is a commonly hypothesized association between a child having a disability and being abused or neglected, few studies exist in this area. Almost totally lacking are well-controlled, whole-population studies of this association for clearly defined subtypes of disability, specifically ASD. In this paper, we describe how secondary data on children with ASD will be linked to other, existing databases to address issues of child abuse and neglect. Our approach is using data from well-documented ASD cases of eight-year-olds in the Tennessee Autism and Developmental Disabilities Monitoring (ADDM) Network database; these children are then matched to comparison cases in the Tennessee Department of Children's Services (TDCS) database. Our ultimate goal is to create an analysis dataset, using ADDM and TDCS data, to examine potential differences in prevalence rates, dispositions, and correlates of abuse among children with ASD. We show the potential of this approach by presenting preliminary findings from a large, population-level study of children with ASD (N = 358) and matched controls.

1. INTRODUCTION

Although there is a commonly hypothesized association between disability status and a child's propensity for abuse and neglect, few well-controlled whole-population studies examine this issue. Even fewer studies exist that examine the prevalence, nature, or correlates of child abuse for clearly defined subtypes of disability, specifically autism spectrum disorder

(ASD). Historically, estimates of increased risk of child abuse among disability populations have been obtained via extrapolation from highly selected groups to national populations (see Sullivan & Knutson, 2000; Spencer et al., 2005). More generally, however, most state agencies charged with investigating allegations of maltreatment (e.g., abuse and neglect) do not have embedded methods for documenting disability status in their child protection records (Sullivan & Knutson, 2000).

An additional complicating factor involves the definition of disability. Across state systems of care and research studies, disability definitions varied widely, limiting our understanding of the exact nature of maltreatment concerns within more specific developmental disability groups (Spencer et al., 2005). Yet it is quite possible that the factors associated with maltreatment for children with intellectual and developmental disabilities (ID/DD) may vary substantially based on the type of disability. One might expect, for example, difference in the prevalence rates of abuse may occur when children have Down syndrome or fragile X syndrome, fetal alcohol syndrome, learning disability, and ASD. So too many different disabilities differ in their type of maltreatment (Duan et al., 2015; Hershkowitz, Lamb, & Horowitz, 2007).

Children with ASD may be particularly prone to child abuse and neglect. There have been numerous hypotheses offered as to why children with ASD may potentially experience maltreatment at higher levels than children without ASD (Berg, Shiu, Msall, & Acharya, 2015; Duan et al., 2015; Howlin & Clements, 1995; Mandell, Walrath, Manteuffel, Sgro, & Pinto-Martin, 2005). Possible risk factors include:

- significant challenging behaviors;
- increased levels of caregiver depression, anxiety, and stress even relative to other ID/DD populations;
- reported lower levels of psychosocial and familial support and social isolation;
- potent impairments related to social interaction and communication skills;
- complex cognitive impairments for some children; and
- adaptive behavior deficits that require increased levels of caregiver dependence.

While it is logical to hypothesize that such factors could lead ASD populations to be at elevated risk for maltreatment, others have suggested that it may be an oversimplification to treat ASD itself as a risk factor for maltreatment (see Mandell et al., 2005). Instead, more specific child, family, and social factors may be more powerfully associated with maltreatment across this heterogeneous grouping of children.

To date, there have been relatively few whole-population studies of ID/DD and maltreatment, with existing studies including small and poorly defined groups of children with ASD. However, in one study of a nonclinical population utilizing school and child protection records in Nebraska, Sullivan and Knutson (2000) found a strong association between disability and maltreatment, with rates of abuse over three times more likely in children with versus without disabilities (31.0%–9%, respectively). This seminal work is often cited as the primary data when discussing increased levels of maltreatment in ID/DD populations, with subsequent works also discussing high rates of maltreatment (see Spencer et al., 2005; Duan et al., 2015).

In more closely examining this study, however, the evidence is unclear for increased rates of abuse among children with ASD. Sullivan and Knutson (2000) actually had only a small number of children with autism in their sample, with a prevalence rate of ASD (0.40%) that is quite disproportionate to current estimated prevalence statistics (1.47%). Further, this small group of children with ASD actually demonstrated comparable levels of maltreatment (9%) to the population of children without disabilities.

An additional whole-population study in the United Kingdom again documented that children with ID/DD were at increased risk of registration within the child protection system. But in a similar way to Sullivan and Knutson (2000), Spencer, Wallace, Sundrum, Bacchus, and Logan (2006) also documented that the pattern of registration varied substantially by the specific disability condition. There was a strong association with maltreatment for severe challenging behaviors (e.g., conduct disorder) and learning difficulties. Children with ASD, as defined by this study, did not demonstrate increased rates of maltreatment. Despite a whole population methodology, this study failed to identify/include a sufficient number of children with ASD (0.3%), thus, leaving questions of just how representative that study's subjects with ASD were to the overall ASD population in the United Kingdom.

In summary, despite the commonly offered hypothesis that children with ASD are at greater risk for maltreatment than other children, few studies using population level data support this hypothesis (Spencer et al., 2006; Sullivan & Knutson, 2000). Under closer examination, the existing studies often have few subjects with ASD (making analyses difficult); the participants with ASD that they do have are likely only a subset of the wider population of children with ASD; and studies do not always find higher rates of abuse among these children. But given the increased interest in ASD now and growing number of children with the disorder (CDC, 2017), it is important to understand the nature and scale of maltreatment for individuals with ASD in order to realize systems of care that can adequately serve them. In this project, then, we attempt to generate evidence regarding the prevalence of maltreatment among a large, population-level sample of children meeting well-defined and established criteria for ASD.

At this point, then, the consensus supports the conclusion that children with ID/DD are at increased risk for maltreatment (American Academy of Pediatrics, 2001; Crosse, Kaye, & Ratnofsky, 1992; Fisher, Hodapp, & Dykens, 2008; Sullivan & Knutson, 2000; Wyckoff, 2011). But the association between ASD and maltreatment is less well documented. Further, while previous work has linked educational classifications of developmental disabilities to child maltreatment concerns (Sullivan & Knutson, 2000), larger epidemiological studies are more limited, specifically in addressing ASD within child protection systems.

The question of identifying the prevalence of maltreatment in an ASD population is, on the face of it, straightforward. It seems that one can simply obtain data addressing the question to then calculate the prevalence of ASD and maltreatment. However, there are substantial definitional and methodological issues that are not easily resolved (American Academy of Pediatrics, 2001; Fisher et al., 2008; Govindshenoy & Spencer, 2007).

2. INTRODUCING A NEW RESEARCH STRATEGY

For the last decade, our research group at the Vanderbilt Kennedy Center has been using large public health datasets and surveys to investigate morbidity and mortality and family issues associated with ID/DD. Although the rationale for using secondary data was presented in an earlier issue of *IRRDD* (see Urbano, Beck, & Stephens, 2013), we highlight that there are both pros and cons to using secondary methodology to study child abuse/neglect among children with ASD.

While one could generate an almost endless list, five major benefits accrue from using secondary data to study issues in ID/DD. First, large-scale secondary datasets allow for a wider perspective, a widening of what might be called the domains of information available. In our work so far, we have used information from statewide birth, death, marriage, divorce, electronic medical records and hospital discharge records. These records are incredibly rich in the information collected. In many disability conditions, for example, questions arise concerning birth status. Are, for example, children with autism more likely to be born prematurely or at low birth weights? What is the effect of having a child with disabilities—or with Down syndrome, autism, or another specific condition—on rates of divorce? These types of questions can now receive research attention.

Second, such research attention can include larger numbers of children and their families, as well as participants who more often represent the larger population. To give one example, our initial study of divorce in Down syndrome (Urbano & Hodapp, 2007) included 647 families of children with Down syndrome. In addition—and unlike many studies which use clients or other samples of convenience—the study included families of children with Down syndrome born throughout Tennessee. As a result, the sample included children who were of lower income and/or minority groups, families that oftentimes are lacking in disability studies.

Third, studies using secondary datasets are oftentimes less costly (Hodapp, Goldman, & Urbano, 2013). As sociologists have noted from the 1960s forward (e.g., Glaser, 1963), the costs of research mostly relate to the collection of data. Research assistants, recruitment visits, payments to participants—all require substantial outlays of money. In contrast, when using statewide administrative data, the costs of collecting, say, birth records, have already been paid by various state departments (e.g., Department of Health or Division of Child and Youth Services), by hospitals, or by other entities. Granted, such datasets are not always free—the main impediment being the form in which such data exist and the need to clean the data.

Fourth—and related—is the issue of linkage. The main power of secondary datasets arises from linking within and between datasets. For example, our earlier work linked within birth records by combining the subsequent birth records from the same mother. Thus, Burke, Hodapp, and Urbano (2011) were able to examine individual mothers' reproductive history—do, for example, mothers have one or more subsequent children after the birth of their offspring with Down syndrome? Other work combined across different types of records, for example, the divorce study noted above (Urbano & Hodapp, 2007). Increasingly, such linkages are becoming easier, with the implementation of such relatively easy-to-use data linkage packages such as freely extensible biomedical record linkage (Christen, 2008).

Fifth, a major benefit of secondary data analysis procedures involves analyses over large blocks of time. By using already collected data, one can create profiles of, say, hospitalization or child abuse or educational history, each over larger time spans. In contrast, a single study that collected its own data is often limited to a 3-year or 5-year span. At times, grants can be renewed to allow for a doubling or tripling of the study's time span. In contrast, however, administrative records often go back 20 or more years, allowing for a much longer term of analysis.

Against these many benefits of secondary analysis, there are several drawbacks. Again, the list of characteristics could extend for longer, but here we focus on two of the "cons" of secondary analysis. The first—the idea that such analyses are performed on "somebody else's data" (SED)—has several implications. The second more relates to issues found within the ASD population itself.

The problem of SED extends in several directions. First, one must consider the variables themselves. Most often, the datasets of interest were originally designed for purposes related to billing (e.g., hospital discharge), demographics (e.g., birth), or public health (birth or death records). As such, they were not designed for the study at hand. As a result, the researcher might like to have asked one or more extra questions. But in the years—even decades—after the data have been collected, no opportunity exists for adding in extra variables.

Beyond what gets asked, the SED problem also relates to how the question(s) got asked. Often, there will be only a single question for some construct (say, depression) that might have benefited from a longer questionnaire. At other points, one is using a question beyond its original intent. To give one hypothetical example, one might want to extrapolate from when and how many prenatal visits the mother had (from the birth records) to her degree of conscientiousness. While such a jump has some face validity, it does nevertheless require a juxtaposition that may or may not be defensible.

Ultimately, the SED problem concerns the quality of the data collected. To what extent can—and should—one accept these data? To many researchers not steeped in secondary datasets, the answer to this question is strictly negative. To these researchers, one must have collected the data oneself in order for that data to be of high quality. In contrast, secondary data researchers have found that the answer must be more nuanced. Specifically, some questions, or areas of question, are fairly reliable, whereas others are not. In analyzing information from statewide birth records, most information about the mother (age, education level, prenatal visits) seems fairly accurate, most information about the father is not

(DiGiuseppe, Aron, Ranbom, Harper, & Rosenthal, 2002; Kirby, 2001). Evaluation of the hospital discharge diagnoses index and the birth certificate as sources of information on birth defects (Hexter et al., 1990).

An additional SED problem relates to autism. As noted in the studies above, few records of studies have provided sophisticated measures of autism. In most of these studies, one does not even know how the child with autism received that diagnosis. This state of affairs differs greatly from the use of the Autism Diagnostic Observation Schedule (ADOS; Lord et al., 2012), Autism Diagnostic Interview (ADI; Rutter, Le Couteur, & Lord, 2003), and other "gold standard" measures within the autism community. In short, one must appreciate that the SED status of secondary datasets will also relate to disability diagnosis, in this case whether the child does or does not truly have ASD.

Given this pattern of pros and cons, many reviews of how, exactly, to perform large-scale, secondary dataset studies have appeared in the literature. A detailed description of the methods used in a real-world study of child outcomes was presented from the Maternal Infant Health Worker (MIHOW) intervention program (Elkins, Aguinaga, Clinton-Selin, Clinton, & Gotterer, 2013). Data on participants in MIHOW were linked to birth vital records to assess the birth outcomes for children of mothers participating in the program.

Both deterministic and probabilistic linking procedures were used to link MIHOW program records and vital birth records to assess birth outcomes. Consistent with the finding of an empirical comparison of deterministic and probabilistic linkage (Gomatam, Carter, Ariet, & Mitchell, 2002) the resulting deterministically and probabilistically linked, analysis dataset produced almost exactly the same results.

The R (R Core Team, 2016) computer programs used for doing the linkage were presented in appendices to that Chapter In addition, Hodapp, Urbano, and So (2006) used linkage and epidemiologic methods to examine outcomes affecting young children and their families.

3. OUR APPROACH

We now explore the application of the epidemiology/linkage methodology our research group has been developing over the last decade to the question: "Are children with ASD at increased risk of experiencing maltreatment?".

We will address three major issues in studies of maltreatment and ASD:

1. How is maltreatment measured?
2. How is disability defined? Specifically, how are cases of ASD identified? and
3. How are cases and comparison groups selected?

3.1 Measurement of Maltreatment

The child welfare system considers two types of maltreatment: abuse and neglect. Abuse is further subdivided into physical, sexual, and emotional (Fisher et al., 2008). Historically, there has not been consistent inclusion of all types of abuse in studies of maltreatment. Indeed, some studies have included one or more (but not all) types of maltreatment; some do not clearly define which types of maltreatment are included or include overlapping types of maltreatment; some have examined abuse categories as predefined by convenience of identification/documentation; and, finally, other studies do not differentiate the type of maltreatment but rather choose to use a global maltreatment category.

Moreover, simple categorization by type often fails to serve as a marker for severity of the maltreatment and by proxy the potential adverse effect. In the current work, we attempt to understand the experiences of children in the child welfare system. For this reason, we included metrics of system-level response rather than predefined heterogeneous categories of maltreatment. We thus assumed that child protective services decisions regarding response to allegations would be highly correlated with potential adverse impact for the child (i.e., children removed from home versus children where only initial concern was noted).

3.2 Tennessee Department of Children's Services Records

Comprehensive administrative records document the processes used to reach a decision regarding an allegation of maltreatment. In the Tennessee Department of Children's Services (TDCS) system, allegations are handled either as an assessment or investigation. Depending on the process applied to an allegation, the disposition of an allegation is recorded in an assessment or investigation dataset (Investigating Maltreatment, 2017).

3.2.1 Assessment

"The Assessment approach seeks to understand the underlying conditions and factors that could jeopardize a child's safety. The focus becomes not just the child but the entire family and its identifiable strengths. By building on those strengths and understanding a family's needs, TDCS can help families avoid the pitfalls that may have previously put their children at risk."

3.2.2 *Investigation*

"Some parents are not able to keep their children safe. For all reports of severe neglect or abuse, a traditional investigation will still take place. Law enforcement will be asked to assist in cases where severe abuse has been reported."

3.2.3 *Decision*

"Allegations brought to the TDCS are resolved with a decision recorded in the TDCS database. For cases processed via the assessment process, the decision is whether or not the family will get services. For cases processed via the investigation process, the allegation is substantiated or not."

3.2.4 *Maltreatment*

"As an operational definition of maltreatment, the TDCS recorded decisions of 'service required' or 'allegation substantiated' were classified as instances of maltreatment" (Your Client's Rights, 2017).

3.3 ASD Classification

In the datasets documenting maltreatment reports, specific disabilities are not necessarily used or included (Spencer et al., 2005). Even when included, ID/DD may be defined by the federal disability categories (http://idea.ed.gov/), medical diagnoses (DSM-5), or locally defined administrative codes (https://www.tn.gov/didd/). Regardless of the classification system used, the task of assigning disability categories to cases by TDCS may be left to individuals with little or no training in developmental disabilities. Rather than depending on a classification of ASD by TDCS, we propose to use the classification of ASD made by the Autism and Developmental Disabilities Monitoring (ADDM) project.

3.4 Study Samples

Population-based studies have the greatest potential for determining unbiased, accurate estimates of the risk of maltreatment. However, most studies of maltreatment use samples of convenience obtained from abuse registries, clinical settings, or children receiving special education services (Berg et al., 2015; Duan et al., 2015; Howlin & Clements, 1995; Mandell et al., 2005).

Such studies using samples of convenience are unlikely to be representative of the general population and thus introduces unknown levels of bias. For example, cases from a clinical setting may not include children and families who are not able to receive services within these systems of care or may disproportionately represent severe cases/presentations. As a result, only the most extreme degrees of maltreatment may be captured. Although methods like capture/recapture analyses can be used to estimate the number of missing cases, such analyses are almost never done.

In a comprehensive review of the research literature, Govindshenoy and Spencer (2007) reviewed population-based studies of the relationship between abuse and disability (Table 1). They used strict criteria for the studies included in the review. Only cohort, case–control or cross-sectional studies of children under 18 years of age were considered. The studies needed to report empirical evidence of the association of maltreatment and disability. Further, risk estimates needed to be reported as odds ratios with 95% confidence intervals. Of 47 papers reviewed, only 4 met their strict selection criteria (Brown, Cohen, Johnson, & Salzinger, 1998; Sidebotham & Heron, 2006; Spencer et al., 2005; Vizcarra, Cortés, Bustos, Alarcón, & Munoz, 2001).

Each study included in the review was rated on five criteria with a maximum score of 10.

1. Sample size: adequate for all aspects of analysis = 2; adequate for most of analyses = 1; inadequate = 0.
2. Attrition rate: $<20\% = 2$; $\geq 20\% = 0$.
3. Confounding variables accounted for: adequate = 2; partially = 1; not accounted for = 0.
4. Exposure definition (disability): well defined = 2; partially defined = 1; poorly defined = 0.
5. Outcome definition (abuse): well defined = 2; partially defined = 1; poorly defined = 0.

Unfortunately, no study obtained a score of 10. If we consider just two of the criteria as the absolute minimum for an adequate study—the existence of a well-defined definition of disability and a well-defined definition of abuse—only two of the studies met criteria (Brown et al. 1998; Spencer et al. 2005). Even then, the Brown et al., study defined "handicapped child" based on parent report of children receiving school-based special education services).

Table 1 Scoring of Studies Using Govindshenoy and Spencer's (2007) Criteria

		Scoring Variables					
Study	**Study Type**	**Sample Size**	**Attrition Rate**	**Confounding Variables Accounted For**	**Exposure Defined (Disability)**	**Outcome Definition (Abuse)**	**Total**
Spencer et al. (2005)	Retrospective birth cohort N = 119,729	1	2	1	2	2	8
Sidebotham and Heron (2006)	Prospective birth cohort N = 14,893	2	2	1	1	2	8
Vizcarra et al. (2001)	Cross-sectional survey N = 422	2	2	0	0	2	6
Brown et al. (1998)	Longitudinal N = 644	1	0	0	2	2	5

4. METHODS

After obtaining approval for this research project from the Vanderbilt University Institutional Review Board, data requests were submitted to the three entities responsible for managing and sharing data they collect. These data custodians have established protocols for releasing data for research purposes. The requested data were provided by the three data custodiansthe ADDM project, TDCS, and the Tennessee Department of Health (TDH). One of the more difficult and time-consuming tasks in research using existing datasets is actually obtaining electronic copies of the needed datasets. Fortunately, for this study, we were able to build on well-established, long-standing collaborations and working relationships with the agencies acting as the custodians of the datasets.

Several factors helped to facilitate the process of obtaining the desired datasets. First, the Principal Investigator (PI) for the ADDM project (ZW) is a "key study" investigator on this study. Also, ZW was able to obtain permission from the Centers for Disease Control and Prevention (CDC) to use the TN ADDM data for this study. Second, another ADDM collaborator (RE) has a strong working relationship with TDCS, which facilitated obtaining their dataset.

Finally, TDH had already provided the 2006 birth records to the ADDM project and subsequently gave permission to use the dataset for the current investigation. The TDH birth dataset was used to determine the number and demographics of the 2006 births in potential surveillance counties contiguous with Davidson County (Nashville, TN) and was used to plan the ADDM surveillance project. Ultimately, electronic datasets for children born in 2006 were obtained from all three entities.

Once permission was obtained and the custodian entity extracted from the requested data, the datasets were transferred to a secure, limited access computer facility at the university. In such an arrangement, the data are protected by multiple layers of physical and electronic security. First, only three non-data center university employees are allowed physical access to the secure computer with the data. Second, there is no direct access to the secure server from outside of the data center, with a gateway computer providing a bridge between the data center and the outside world. This indirect access pathway is controlled by a set of public/private encryption key pairs. Access to the encryption keys is tightly controlled. Data center security personnel control the installation of the encryption keys. Third, the entire disk storage on the secure server is encrypted. Thus, the data on the secure server cannot be accessed without the key phrase originally used to encrypt the disks.

4.1 Dataset Used to Study Maltreatment and ASD

To study ASD and maltreatment, data were collected from the three data sources (ADDM, Birth vital records, and TDCS). By linking data on individuals across these three datasets, a single dataset can be created with information on ASD, allegations of maltreatment, processing of the allegations by TDCS, and the TDCS determined maltreatments status. The specific information provided by each data source is detailed in the following sections.

4.2 Tennessee Department of Children's Service (TDCS) Datasets

4.2.1 TDCS Workflow

During the study time period, the TDCS employed differential response for child protective services. As an approach to structuring child protective services, differential response is based on the premise that not all referrals to child protective services require the so-called "traditional response" of investigation as a criminal matter (Department of Health and Human Services, Children's Bureau, 2014). In this way, differential response is premised on the idea that different initial interventions are more likely to be helpful in certain circumstances and/or for certain referrals. For example, it might be helpful to respond to a report of inadequate supervision differently than to a report of severe physical or sexual abuse.

Although jurisdictions vary regarding how differential response is implemented, in general, there are two broad categories of differential responses: Investigation responses (called "Investigations" by TDCS) and alternative responses (called "Assessments" by TDCS). In TDCS and elsewhere, Investigations and Assessments occur after initial referrals are made via the TDCS child abuse hotline or other direct contacts. A triage process, involving a safety and risk assessment, is used to determine whether to refer a potential case to the Investigation or Assessment response. Potential cases may also be screened out (i.e., not requiring action by TDCS), referred to alternative community resources (e.g., food stamps), or referred to a special investigations unit (e.g., perpetrator is in a professional role such as school teacher, coach, or foster parent).

It is important to note that differential response approaches to child protective services, TDCS's included, do not necessarily follow a simple linear referral-assessment/investigation-decision set of steps. After an initial processing of a referral case, new information may dictate the need to adjust the system's response. For example, a call to a child abuse hotline due to concerns about unsanitary living conditions might initially be triaged to an Assessment response. But with further examination, the TDCS worker may uncover potentially dangerous parental substance abuse or other concerns; at that point, the referral would be changed to an Investigation response.

The five datasets provided to the study team by the TDCS (hotline, assessments, investigations, removals, exits) represent major points at which individuals interact with the system. Three of these datasets—Hotline, Investigations, and Assessments—document initial contacts with the system and differential responses to that initial contact. In the Removals dataset are recorded all of the cases that are investigated or assessed and determined to require removal of the child to the custody of TDCS. From among those cases in the Removals dataset, those completing the required TDCS interventions are recorded in the Exit dataset.

The two datasets provided by TDCS will be the focus of this study: (1) Investigations and (2) Assessments. The Investigations and Assessment datasets record cases that have been triaged for further action and reflect important responses to initial reports of maltreatment. Investigations or assessments result in a decision about the allegation.

4.3 Autism and Developmental Disabilities Monitoring Data

4.3.1 ADDM Project

ASD is a relatively common disorder associated with enormous costs to individuals, families, communities, and systems of care, both in terms of dollars and human experience (Ammerman, Van Hasselt, Hersen, McGonigle, & Lubetsky, 1989). The estimated prevalence of ASD has increased dramatically over the past three decades. Rigorous epidemiological and surveillance methodologies have identified several factors contributing to increases in ASD over this timeframe (Wingate et al., 2014). However, significant scientific uncertainty remains regarding the underlying causes of these substantial increases in identification. Due to the significant lifespan medical, educational, and service needs of this population, accurate prevalence estimates are essential in order to address the public health issues associated with ASD.

Given the complexities of accurately identifying this behaviorally defined disorder and ascertaining large enough samples to understand variability across important subgroups, both survey methodologies and simple aggregate special education reports are not adequate for understanding ASD prevalence and prevalence changes (Christensen, 2016). In this capacity, the CDC ADDM network and affiliated surveillance partners offer substantial benefits. Specifically, ADDM and its partners are uniquely positioned to provide the most scientifically rigorous prevalence estimates of ASD in the United States. In addition, ADDM and partners can provide additional crucial information regarding the important characteristics underlying this complex, heterogeneous disorder (i.e., co-occurring conditions, age of evaluation/diagnosis, level of functioning) and its accurate identification (i.e., disparities in gender, race/ethnicity).

4.3.2 ADDM Methodology

Unlike most previous studies, ADDM network methodology does not rely on professional or family reporting of diagnoses or classification to determine ASD case status. Instead, two active surveillance phases are employed before ASD status is assigned, including 1) abstraction and 2) clinician review. In an effort to "cast the widest net," individual ADDM sites request both educational and health records for a particular birth cohort (i.e., 8-year-olds) in a predetermined surveillance area. Education records are identified from eligibility classifications in special education and health records from International Classification of Diseases, Ninth Revision (ICD-9) billing codes for select childhood disabilities or psychological conditions.

Due to the wide range of professionals that are involved in screening and assessing developmental concerns, records are requested from many providers. Among those from whom records are requested are psychologists, neurologists, developmental pediatricians, physical therapists, occupational therapists, and speech/language pathologists. In many cases, the request of records requires formal data use agreements between the ADDM network site and the source.

Once the records have been procured, a team of reviewers examines each record. After potential cases have been identified, qualifying evaluations are screened for specific social communication and restrictive and repetitive behavior "triggers." These include such issues as the child not initiating interactions with others, preferring to play alone or engage in solitary activities, or receiving a documented ASD diagnosis.

Once these triggers are noted, the next step in the process begins. Specifically, once triggers are found, all available records on that child are abstracted and compiled. The compiled, de-identified record is then sent to a trained clinician to code based on DSM-5 autism criteria. Case definition is met if a child qualifies for DSM-5 criteria based off of behavioral descriptions in qualifying reports from birth to age eight.

For this study, the Tennessee ADDM site employed a team of six abstractors who were bachelor's level research assistants with experience in ASD. The clinician review team consisted of four master's and doctorate level clinicians with extensive knowledge in ASD. All personnel were provided initial training through staff at the CDC. In order to achieve and maintain the reliability of the ADDM network and methodology, the Tennessee site manager conducted ongoing quality assurance and control activities for both abstractors and clinician reviewers. For the abstraction team, after reaching initial reliability on CDC practice records, at least 10% of local files were reviewed and assessed for content and the decision to abstract. Clinician reviewers established initial reliability with a set of records provided by the CDC; then internal reliability was established at the site with a set of ten local records. In order to guard against "drift" in inter-coder reliability, continued reliability was maintained by reviewing every 10th record.

In the Tennessee ADDM project, the surveillance area for 8-year-old children included 11 counties. These comprised the counties of Bedford, Cheatham, Davidson, Dickson, Marshall, Maury, Montgomery, Rutherford, Robertson, Williamson, and Wilson. As shown in Fig. 1, these 11 counties

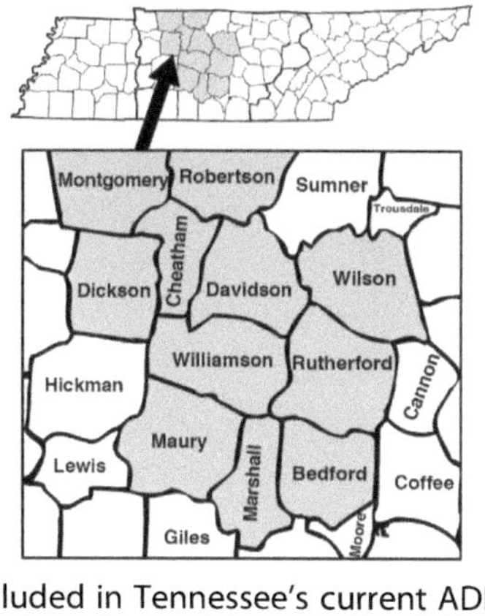

Figure 1 Counties included in Tennessee's current ADDM surveillance cycle.

represent a contiguous geography in the middle Tennessee region. According to the latest post-census estimates, a population of 23,968 children were born in 2006 (2014 surveillance) in this area.

In addition to having sufficient numbers of children to allow for analyses, this 11-county area was selected to allow the potential capture of information about children among particularly vulnerable and high-risk groups. This area encompasses a mix of primarily metropolitan counties (Marshall County was the only micropolitan county) with substantial variation in socioeconomic status (median household income range: $39,635–$91,146). Further, this grouping of counties includes the counties of the middle Tennessee region with the most racial/ethnic diversity. In terms of representation to the state of Tennessee (17% Black or African-American, 4.9% Hispanic or Latino, 1.7% Two or more Races, 0.4% American Indian or Alaska 0.1% Native Hawaiian and Other Pacific Islander), 8-year-old estimates suggest fairly comparable representation within this catchment, with slight overrepresentation of Hispanic/Latino individuals. County-based median household income for the middle Tennessee catchment is slightly above that for the state ($44,140); some 17.3% of the Tennessee population is estimated to be below the poverty line with 14.7% represented in the current catchment.

4.3.3 ADDM Data Sources

In addition to its size and demographic diversity, the selected surveillance area also allows for the immediate availability of large networked data systems. These systems provide rapid access to a large percentage of the targeted medical and educational records, including overrepresented populations of interest (e.g., primary systems serving children with ASD/ID). Specifically, Vanderbilt's Mid-South Clinical Data Research Network and Department of Educational and Statewide Student Management System as a core infrastructure and foundation were used for access, request, and data sources. These record infrastructures allowed for almost immediate health source access to records of an estimated 65% of our surveillance area across years, as well as educational eligibility (Part B & C) assessment data through public schools for all children within the proposed geography. Importantly, these systems did not simply represent administrative sources of data, but data warehouses where relevant supporting documentation also resides (i.e., primary evaluation/assessment reports).

Additional health record information was also available on the majority of these children. Specifically, Vanderbilt's health care system includes an affiliated clinical electronic health record infrastructure, known as StarPanel, explicitly designed to speed medical and public health surveillance activities and research activities. StarPanel includes almost two decades of longitudinal data from nearly 2.5 million patients. Currently, Vanderbilt is funded by the Patient Centered Outcomes Research Institute (PCORI) as the leader of a Mid-South Clinical Data Research Network aimed at synthesizing these records for numerous public health surveillance and clinical research activities. The Mid-South Clinical Data Research Network, which includes special emphasis on accessing rural and urban patients, encompasses an electronic health record capture system and data extraction tools that presently include all Vanderbilt University Health System (VUHS) and local partner site records. Together, these sources of data cover 2.5 million individuals and over 1 million active patients. For the 2006 birth year surveillance in the ADDM catchment area, existing medical records were available for 18,436 children.

Additional information was also available. As the VUHS and partner sites include a robust array of hospitals, clinics, and home health services, we were able to access health information from the Monroe Carell, Jr. Children's Hospital, Stallworth Rehabilitation Hospital, and approximately 100 primary care and specialty practices throughout the region. Importantly, this health system includes the Center for Child Development within the Division of Developmental Medicine, the Vanderbilt Bill Wilkerson Center, and Child and Adolescent Psychiatry Services. The Center for Child Development within the Division of Developmental Medicine is the largest tertiary developmental and behavioral pediatric assessment center in the state of Tennessee and the primary center in this regard within middle TN.

Some 6989 children received developmental evaluation services from psychologists, developmental pediatricians, psychiatrists, and nursing providers in 2016 (4188 new patient visits, 2801 returns). A majority of these evaluations were specific to concerns about ASD, ID, and related developmental disabilities (1229 with primary ASD related ICD9 code). The Vanderbilt Bill Wilkerson Center is a well-known communication disorders center, including over 100 audiologists, speech-language pathologists, educational providers, occupational therapists, physical therapists, and social workers. These service providers care for an estimated 350 children with ASD per year (primarily under age 8). Vanderbilt's Child and Adolescent Psychiatry services care for an estimated 1750 unique children per year across outpatient, inpatient, consultative, and school-based mental health services.

All of these service entities, in addition to children served through Vanderbilt's hospitals, pediatric primary care clinics (estimated 32,500 children), as well as affiliated specialty clinics and partners in our region, have medical records currently available for ADDM surveillance activities within the Mid-South Clinical Data Research Network.

In addition, the Vanderbilt Kennedy Center (VKC)/Treatment and Research Institute for Autism Spectrum Disorders (TRIAD) provides services to a vast number of children through a variety of clinical research protocols (e.g., genetics consortium projects, intervention protocols, pharmacological interventions). Many protocols provide aspects of clinical care, including developmental evaluations. For the past 5 years, TRIAD-affiliated protocols have asked parents for appropriate consent for placement of such evaluation records into their child's medical electronic health record for care coordination. These families have also been approached regarding enrollment in active IRB approved research registries. The current TRIAD registry alone has 2646 participants, with 70 represented from our 2006 8-year-old surveillance areas.

To identify those children with an educational (but not medical) diagnosis of ASD, the Tennessee Department of Education (TN DOE) provided support and a formal memo of understanding, granting access to appropriate educational records in the Statewide Student Management System (SSMS). The SSMS is a comprehensive, state provided, web-based electronic student information system for school districts to facilitate local, state, and federal reporting requirements with additional local functionality features. The primary component of this TN DOE system that relates to our proposed work is the EasyIEP. EasyIEP is an Individualized Educational Program (IEP) writer and census reporting tool for special education. The EasyIEP tool stores an individual student's IEP and documents related to special education eligibility. Through our agreement with the TN DOE, we were able to obtain a list of all students in our surveillance area born in 2006 with a current special education classification. In order to access individual student files, each of the 14 public school districts within our 11-county surveillance area was approached. As of June 2017, 13 of these districts have agreed to participate.

4.4 Tennessee Department of Health—Birth Vital Records Dataset

The ADDM surveillance also aimed to pay special attention to improved understanding of ASD and ID within vulnerable populations, including children in state custody and children encountering the juvenile justice system. Past work on the prevalence of youth with psychiatric disorders in the juvenile justice system and in state custody (e.g., foster/adoptive placements) has consistently documented high rates of behavioral challenges. However, several methodological hurdles have limited understanding of the prevalence of children with ASD and ID within these care systems. Specifically, such investigations have often relied on reporter and/or survey strategies, focused on selected subsamples of convenience, and relied on small sample sizes (Cheely et al., 2012).

We have explicitly partnered with TDCS and the Director of Vanderbilt's Center for Excellence in State Custody (COE) to access data for children removed from the home or encountering the juvenile justice system. As a part of a statewide network funded under an agreement with the state, the Vanderbilt COE endeavors to improve public health by enhancing the quality of services provided to children in or at risk of entering the Tennessee child welfare or juvenile justice systems. Children and families involved with these systems are much more likely to have developmental, physical, or psychiatric disabilities, including ASD/ID (Spencer et al., 2005). The Vanderbilt COE provides case consultation and case review, psychological testing, psychiatric evaluation, and medication management to these children. We will access source records available through these services for health source surveillance.

Study Datasets—The variables contained in each of the study datasets are presented in Tables 2–4.

4.4.1 ADDM Dataset

All cases processed by the ADDM project (N = 582) were included in their dataset. Each record contained a unique tracking identification number. Child demographic information included first, middle, and last name, gender, and date of birth. Location information included street address, city, zip code, and county. The results of the review process were recorded in three variables—Autism status (AU) (Confirmed Case, Suspected Case, Pending, Disqualified After Review, Borderline or Mild ID, did not qualify Not Abstracted, did not qualify After Review); Cerebral Palsy status (CP) (Confirmed, Did not qualify); and Intellectual Disability status (ID) (Confirmed, Did not qualify, Did not qualify IQ $>$ 70). Confirmed cases of autism were included in the study (N = 358).

4.4.2 Tennessee Department of Children's Services Datasets

Each TDCS dataset provided demographic information—child first and last name, child date of birth, sex, race—and location information—child

Table 2 Information Exported From the Autism and Developmental Disabilities Monitoring Database

Variable Name	Variable Description
Trackingid	Unique case identifier
AU	Autism status (CONFIRMED CASE, SUSPECTED CASE, PENDING, DISQUALIFIED AFTER REVIEW, Borderline or MILD ID, Did not qualify NOT ABSTRACTED, Did not qualify AFTER REVIEW)
CP	Cerebral Palsy (CONFIRMED, Did not qualify)
ID	Intellectual Disability (CONFIRMED, Did not qualify, Did not qualify IQ>70)
lastname	Child last name
firstname	Child first name
middle	Child middle name
sex	Gender (1 = Male 2 = Female)
dob	Child date of birth (yyyy-mm-dd)
address1	Street address
address2	Apt/Lot#
city	City name
zip	5-digit US zipcode (#####)
county	County name

address, city, and state (see Table 2). The demographic variables were used to link cases in the ADDM dataset and the Comparison group cases with cases in the TDCS datasets. The unique variables in the Assessment and Investigation datasets are described in Tables 3 and 4.

4.4.3 TN Department of Health Birth Vital Records Dataset

The birth vital records dataset contains over 400 individual data elements. For the current study, demographic and locations information were extracted from the birth dataset (Table 5). The specific data elements that permitted selecting control cases and linking the controls to the TDCS datasets are listed in the "Birth Data (Comparison)" column in Table 5.

4.4.4 Variables Used in Record Linkage

Record linkage is the process used to find records from one dataset that match records in a second dataset. For this study, ADDM and birth datasets will be linked to the TDCS Assessment and Investigation datasets. The resulting four linked datasets will be ADDM_Assessment, ADDM_Investigation, Comparison_Assessment, and Comparison_Investigation.

Table 3 Tennessee Department of Children's Services ASSESSMENT Dataset Fields

Variable Name	Description
assessment_date	Assessment Date – YYYY-MM-DD
Allegation	ABANDONMENT: Deliberate absence of the parent or other caretaker for an extended period with no plan or provision for the child's care. ABUSEDEATH: Any child death caused by abuse, any unexplained death of a child when the cause of death is unknown or pending an autopsy report, and any child death caused by abuse resulting from the parent or caretaker's failure to stop another person's direct action that resulted in the death of the child. DRUGEXPOSEDCHILD: Any person under the age of 18 who has been exposed to or is at risk of exposure to a drug or chemical substance that could adversely affect the child's physical, mental or emotional functioning or who has a parent/caregiver that uses drugs or chemical substances that impacts or is at risk of impacting their ability to adequately care for the child. DRUGEXPOSEDINFANT: No longer in use. Replaced by more inclusive Drug Exposed Child. EDUCATIONALNEGLECT: Repeated failure of the parent or caretaker to meet the child's educational needs. ENVIRONMENTALNEGLECT: A living situation either inside or outside the residence that is dangerous or unhealthy. LACKOFSUPERVISION: Failure to provide adequate supervision that results in harm or significant risk of harm, by a parent or other caretaker, who is able to do so. MEDICALMALTREATMENT: A situation in which a child does not receive adequate health care, resulting in actual or potential harm. NEGLECTDEATH: Any child death caused by neglect and any child death caused by neglect resulting from the parent or caretaker's failure to stop another person's direct action that resulted in the death of the child NUTRITIONALNEGLECT: A parent or caretaker's failure to provide adequate nutrition to a child PHYSICALABUSE: Any non-accidental physical injury or trauma that could cause injury inflicted by a parent, caretaker, relative or any other person who is responsible for the care, supervision, or treatment of the child PSYCHOLOGICALHARM: A repeated pattern of caregiver behavior or extreme incident(s) that convey to children that they are worthless, flawed, unloved, unwanted, endangered or

(Continued)

Table 3 Tennessee Department of Children's Services ASSESSMENT Dataset Fields—cont'd

Variable Name	Description
	only of value in meeting another's needs and may include both abusive acts against a child and failure to act.
	SEXUALABUSE: Child sexual abuse occurs when a child who is under the age of 13 or was under the age of 13 when the abuse occurred or a child is of age 13–18 and is involved in intentional sexual acts that produce sexual arousal and/or gratification for the perpetrator.
Decision	ALLEG INDICATE PERP INDICATE: There is a preponderance of evidence to support that an allegation and alleged perpetrator identified in the report is found to be responsible for the alleged acts.
	ALLEG INDICATE PERP UNFOUND: There is a preponderance of evidence to support an allegation, however the alleged perpetrator identified in the report is found to be responsible for the alleged acts
	ALLEG UNFOUND PERP UNFOUND: There is not a preponderance of evidence to support that an allegation and the alleged perpetrator identified in the report is not found to be responsible for the alleged acts.
	ASSESSMENT, NO SERVICES NEEDED: An assessment is completed and no risk or service needs are identified. There are no concerns regarding the safety of the child(ren).
	SERVICES ACCEPTED: There is a need for services, but there is no immediate threat of harm to the safety of the child or family. These encouraged and voluntary services may be new services or existing services the family is recommended to continue.
	SERVICES REFUSED, SERVICES REQUIRED: There is a need for services, but there is no immediate threat of harm to the safety of the child or family. The encouraged and voluntary services recommended to the family are refused.
	TRIBAL COUNSEL RESPONSIBLE, UNABLE TO COMPLETE: The alleged child victim is under the jurisdiction of tribal authority and DCS has no jurisdiction to complete an investigation.
	ADMINISTRATIVE CLOSURE: Reserved for cases that do not meet criteria for any of the above listed classification options. This occurs when there is no indication for an investigation and a courtesy interview(s) has been conducted, or there are other circumstances which are approved at the discretion of the Director of Investigations, or designee.

Table 4 Tennessee Department of Children's Services INVESTIGATION Dataset Fields

Variable Name	Description
Investigation_date	Investigation date – YYYY-MM-DD
Allegation	See Table 3
Substantiated	No (35,671) Yes (8667)

Table 5 Variables Used to Link ADDM, TDCS, and Birth Vital Records Datasets

ADDM Data	TDCS Data	Birth Data (Comparison)
Primary Linking Variables		
lastname	lastname	lastname
firstname	firstname	firstname
sex	sex	sex
dob	dob	dob
Secondary Linking Variables		
county		county
birth month		birth_month

In performing this linkage, we will be using a particular type of linkage, using four specific pieces of information. The process itself will be "deterministic"—that is, we will look for an exact match across all matching variables. This type of linkage is contrasted to so-called "probabilistic" linking, in which partial or near matches are assigned a value reflecting the degree of agreement. The values from the partial matches are weighted and summed. Scores above determined cutoff value are classified as matches. Those below a lower cutoff value are classified as non-matches. Cases between the low and high cutoff boundaries are ambiguous and set aside for further review if possible. Although the benefits and drawbacks of each type of linkage have long been debated (Hodapp et al., 2013), we felt that our data sources were robust enough to allow for deterministic linkage techniques. Such linkage will be accomplished by examining the four demographic variables that are common to all five datasets—lastname, firstname, sex, and date of birth.

The Comparison dataset will be created in a separate, deterministic linkage process. Birth records from the 11 TN counties in the ADDM surveillance area for the birth year 2006 were matched on keys constructed from county, birth month, and sex. Unique values of keys extracted from the ADDM dataset were used to select Comparison cases from the Birth dataset. The keys variable was created by concatenating county, month of birth, and sex separated by colons e.g., "davidson:07:1." The Comparison group will be selected from the matched birth records by sampling every 10th birth record within the key "county-birth month-sex" groups.

5. RECORD LINKAGE

5.1 Data Cleaning

In preparation for linking the three original datasets to create the final linked dataset, all files were read using the statistical package R (R Core Team, 2016). All files provided by the data custodians were, by agreement, in human readable text using CSV (comma separated variables) formatting. Although CSV text files are not the most information dense option, they do provide just enough structure—variable names and comma delimited data—to be read by most programs (e.g., text editors, Excel, most database programs, and statistical packages). Each data custodian had their own standards for naming variables and formatting dates and text fields. In order to standardize the information in each dataset and facilitate the comparisons between datasets the following procedures were applied to each dataset:

1. Variable names were converted to lower case.
2. Variables were renamed in order to be consistent across datasets. For example, child.last.name was renamed to lastname; street.1 was converted to address1; child.dob to dob; and child.sex to sex.
3. Dates were recoded to the format "YYYY-MM-DD." With this ordering of date elements, it is easy to sort records into chronological order
4. Character variables were converted to lower case.
5. Sex was recoded to Male = 1 and Female = 2.
6. Hyphenated last names were reformatted with no spaces around the "-". Multiple last names without hyphens had hyphens added.
7. Special characters were removed from all character fields (e.g., apostrophes and quotes were replaced with spaces).

5.2 Applied Linkage Methodology

The deterministic linkage process to be used with these data is a highly efficient method of determining exact agreement on a selected set of variables. Prime candidates for linking variables are highly specific identifiers such as social security numbers, medical record numbers, or system-generated unique identifiers. Individuals have one and only one value of these identifiers. Birth records have a birth certificate number, and ADDM records have a tracking id. Unfortunately, none of these high quality linking variables occur in more than one of our datasets. Thus, they cannot be used to link datasets.

Alternatively, combinations of less unique variables such as last name, first name, and date of birth may be used as linking variables. For the record linkages needed in this study, key variables were created using combinations last name, first name, date of birth, sex, and county of residence. The set of linked records consists of exact matches on the key variables.

Since deterministic linkage relies on exact matches, the quality of the data used for linking is very important. The three datasets for this study have high quality data on names, date of birth, sex, and county. The data are subjected to multiple edits and review.

Therefore, this study used a deterministic linkage process. Records will be designated as matches if they agree on the "Primary Linking Variables" in Table 5—lastname, firstname, date of birth, and sex.

5.3 Analysis Dataset

The dataset to be used in all analyses will consist of de-identified records from the linked datasets, with eight variables:

1. Group (ADDM/Comparison)
2. Sex (Male/Female)
3. Autism (Yes/No)
4. Allegation ("Yes," "No")
5. Process (ASSESSMENT, INVESTIGATION, NEITHER)
6. Decision ("ADMINISTRATIVE CLOSURE," "ALLEG INDICATE PERP INDICATE," "ALLEG INDICATE PERP UNFOUND,""ALLEG UNFOUND PERP UNFOUND," "NO SERVICES NEEDED," "SERVICES ACCEPTED", "SERVICES REFUSED", "SERVICES REQUIRED," "TRIBAL COUNSEL RESPONSIBLE," "UNABLE TO COMPLETE," "No," "SUBSTANTIATED")
7. Abuse ("Yes" [decision = "ALLEG INDICATE PERP INDICATE," "SERVICES REQUIRED," " SUBSTANTIATED"]/ "NO")
8. Unique id number (programmatically generated and unrelated to any case variables)

6. PRELIMINARY RESULTS

At this time, preliminary results are available on five datasets that will be linked to create an overall analysis dataset.

6.1 ADDM Cases

There are 582 cases in the ADDM dataset with 61.8% (362) classified as confirmed ASD cases. A significantly larger proportion of the ASD cases are male (82.9% vs. 71.9%) (Table 6). Similarly, a large proportion of the ID cases (71.3%) are male, although the proportion of males in the non-ID group is larger (81.8%) (Table 7). Although there is large proportion of cases of ASD and ID in the ADDM group, there is not a significant relationship between ASD and ID. The analysis dataset had 3001 cases. There were 582 (19.4%) cases from the ADDM group and 2419 (80.6%) are from the Comparison group. Thus, the analysis dataset had 4.2 Comparison cases for each ADDM case (Table 8).

6.2 TDCS Cases

There are 28,746 cases in the TDCS datasets, with 51.6% male. A significant proportion of the cases were processed as Investigations (64.5% or 18,541 from among 28,746) compared to 35.5% (10,205/28,746) processed as

Table 6 Proportion of Confirmed ASD Status by Sex in the ADDM Dataset

	Sex		
Autism (Confirmed)	**Male**	**Female**	**Total**
YES	82.9% (300)	17.1% (62)	61.8% (362)
NO	71.9% (161)	28.1% (63)	38.2% (224)
All Cases	78.7% (461)	21.3% (125)	586

$\chi^2(1) = 9.33$ $P = .002$.

Table 7 Proportion of Confirmed Intellectual Disability Status by Sex in the ADDM Dataset

	Sex		
Intellectual Disability (Confirmed)	**Male**	**Female**	**Total**
YES	71.3% (119)	28.7% (48)	71.4% (167)
NO	81.8% (341)	18.2% (76)	28.6% (167)
All Cases	78.8% (460)	21.2% (124)	584

$\chi^2(1) = 7.89$ $P = .005$.

Table 8 Proportion of Confirmed ASD Status by Confirmed Intellectual Disability in the ADDM Dataset

	Intellectual Disability (Confirmed)		
Autism (Confirmed)	**Yes**	**No**	**Total**
Yes	73.4% (265)	26.6% (96)	61.8% (361)
No	68.2% (152)	31.8% (71)	38.2% (223)
All Cases	71.4% (417)	28.6% (167)	584

$\chi^2(1) = 1.86$ $P = .17$.

Assessments. A slightly higher proportion of males (52.5% (5362/10,295)) were processed as Assessments versus being processed as Investigations (51.1% (9472/18,541)) (Table 9). A slightly higher (22.6% vs 21.2%) proportion of cases processed as Assessment are classified as maltreatment (Table 10). Although, given such large numbers, this 0.4% difference is statistically significant; it is not clinically important.

6.3 Birth Cases

Across the 11-county ADDM catchment area, there are 23,968 birth records. The distribution of cases by county in the birth and ADDM datasets are not significantly different. Males make up 51.1% of the cases.

Table 9 TDCS Cases by Processing Type and Sex

	Sex		
Processing Type	**Male**	**Female**	**Total**
Assessment	52.5% (5362)	47.5% (4843)	35.5% (10,205)
Investigation	51.1% (9472)	48.9% (9069)	64.5% (18,541)
All Cases	51.6% (14,834)	48.4% (13,912)	28,746

$\chi^2(1) = 5.53$ $P = .019$.

Table 10 TDCS Cases by Processing Type and Maltreatment

	Maltreatment		
Processing Type	**No**	**Yes**	**Total**
Assessment	77.4% (7932)	22.6% (2316)	35.6% (10,248)
Investigation	78.8% (14,609)	22.1% (3929)	64.4% (18,538)
All Cases	51.6% (14,609)	48.4% (6245)	28,786

$\chi^2(1) = 7.67$ $P = .006$.

Table 11 Number of Cases by County in Birth and ADDM Datasets

	Birth Dataset		ADDM Dataset	
County	**N**	**%**	**N**	**%**
Bedford[a]	706	02.9%	18	03.1%
Blount	0	00.0%	1	00.2%
Cheatham[a]	450	01.9%	12	02.0%
Davidson[a]	9883	41.2%	179	30.5%
Dickson[a]	702	02.9%	20	03.4%
Humphreys	—	—	1	00.2%
Lawrence	—	—	1	0.20%
Lewis	—	—	1	00.2%
Marshall[a]	391	01.6%	13	00.2%
Maury[a]	1080	04.5%	34	05.8%
Montgomery[a]	2561	10.7%	81	13.8%
Robertson[a]	1041	04.3%	17	02.9%
Rutherford[a]	3624	15.1%	90	15.4%
Sumner	—	—	4	00.7%
Williamson[a]	2150	09.0%	63	10.8%
Wilson[a]	1380	05.8%	39	06.7%
Missing	—	—	12	02.0%
Total	23,968			586

[a]Counties in the ADDM catchment area.

Interestingly, there are seven ADDM cases currently living in counties outside the 11-county catchment area. The CDC guidance only requires that a case must have lived in the catchment area at some time during the school year. An additional 12 ADDM cases do not have a county recorded. These will be updated from the address information in ADDM.

Comparison cases will be drawn from the birth dataset based on county, birth month and sex. Since there are seven ADDM cases from four counties outside the original 11-county catchment area, no comparison cases can be found for those cases. Thus, four counties will be added to the subset of counties in the full 2006 birth dataset from which comparison cases will be drawn (Table 11).

7. NEXT STEPS

With the core dataset obtained and preprocessing completed, it will be possible to create an analysis dataset with ADDM and comparison cases linked to TDCS cases. The ADDM to TDCS-linked records will have

Table 12 Analysis Dataset Structure—Groups and Variables

	ADDM			TDCS		
	Autism (Y/N)	Allegation (list)	Allegation_yn (Y/N)	Action_type (Assessment or Investigation)	TDCS Decision (list)A	Abuse (Y/N)
ADDM						
Comparison						

ASD status and TDCS processing and outcome information. The birth to ADDM to TDCS linkage will produce matched comparison cases with their TDCS processing and outcome information. By design, the comparison group has no ASD cases (Table 12).

7.1 Research Questions

The analysis dataset can be used to address three specific research questions. Each question is annotated with the variables that will be used to answer the question.

1. Are children with ASD more likely than comparison children to have an allegation registered with TDCS?

   ASD status comes from the ADDM data. Allegations come from the Assessment and Investigation data. The allegation variable in the Assessment and Investigation data are recoded to allegation_YN (the allegation variable which has multiple values has been coded as Yes/No). ASD status is also coded as Yes/No. The cross-tabulation of ASD and allegation_YN will be used.
2. Given that an allegation has been made with TDCS, are children with ASD processed differently than comparison children?

   The two processes used by TDCS of Assessments and Investigations are recorded in the process_type variable. The cross-tabulation of ASD by process_type will be used.
3. Are children with ASD more likely than comparison children to have a decision recorded by TDCS as maltreatment?

   The decision reached by TDCS is recorded as Yes/No in the variable abuse. The cross-tabulation of ASD status and abuse will be used.

8. DISCUSSION

Past work on the prevalence of ID/DD among youth involved in the child welfare system (e.g., foster/adoptive placements) has consistently documented high rates of maltreatment. Given that 40%–75% of individuals with ASD may also have ID, as well as the fundamental core impairments of the disorder itself, it is likely that these youths would also experience high rates of interaction with the child welfare system. Further, children with ASD have multiple risk factors associated with abuse/maltreatment. It is reasonable to assume that the cumulative effect of such risk factors would result in an increased likelihood of entering the child protection service system and an increased prevalence of maltreatment/neglect.

The two best controlled population studies (Spencer et al., 2006; Sullivan & Knutson, 2000) with small samples of individuals with ASD did not find a difference in the prevalence of maltreatment for youth with ASD as compared to controls without ASD. However, several methodological hurdles have limited our understanding of the prevalence of children with ASD within the child welfare system. Specifically, such investigations have often relied on reporter and/or survey strategies, focused on selected subsamples of convenience, relied on small sample sizes for the target population, and operated with poorly defined categories for the disorder itself.

A process using secondary data may be used to address three methodical issues not addressed in prior studies. First, obtain data on a well-characterized population of eight-year-olds with ASD identified by the Tennessee ADDM project. The CDC ADDM protocol implements a detailed procedure for evaluating existing records to determine cases of ASD. The number of cases of ASD identified in the ADDM catchment area (N = 358) is larger than in any other published population study on maltreatment. Second, use record linkage methods to create datasets combining ADDM, Birth, and TDCS data. Child profiles of cases with and without ASD can be used to characterize the ways in which children were triaged into different tracks in the TDCS system. Third, link a sample of birth records with the same county, birth month, and sex as cases in the ADDM dataset to create a comparison group. This matched group of individuals from the ADDM catchment area provides a baseline for comparing referrals to and outcomes for the cases in the child welfare system.

In summary, secondary data and record linkage can be used to create a combined dataset with variables necessary to test the simple and commonly offered hypothesis that children with ASD are at greater risk for maltreatment than other children based simply on the classification of the disorder itself. Linking additional information from other secondary data to the current datasets will allow further examination of the characteristics within this broad, heterogeneous grouping of ASD. There may be that some children with ASD exhibit increased vulnerability to certain forms of maltreatment, encounters, and outcomes. It is also quite possible that the pathways in response to welfare system encounters differ for some children with ASD based on their characteristics. Future work is needed to more fully understand whether specific characteristics of individuals within and across the autism spectrum are associated with higher rates of encounter, and ultimately to better understand, design, and equip child welfare systems to promote optimal engagement through these systems of care.

ACKNOWLEDGMENTS

Preparation of the chapter was funded in part by the CDC Surveillance Grant (5U53DD001170-02) and the NICHDH U54 grant (HD83211-01A1).

REFERENCES

American Academy of Pediatrics. (2001). Assessment of maltreatment of children with disabilities. *Pediatrics, 108*(2), 508–512.

Ammerman, R. T., Van Hasselt, V. B., Hersen, M., McGonigle, J. J., & Lubetsky, M. J. (1989). Abuse and neglect in psychiatrically hospitalized multihandicapped children. *Child Abuse & Neglect, 13*(3), 335–343.

Berg, K. L., Shiu, C.-S., Msall, M. E., & Acharya, K. (June 1, 2015). Victimization and restricted participation among young people with disabilities in the US child welfare system. *Developmental Medicine & Child Neurology, 57*(6), 564–570. http://dx.doi.org/10.1111/dmcn.12678.

Brown, J., Cohen, P., Johnson, J. G., & Salzinger, S. (November 1998). A longitudinal analysis of risk factors for child maltreatment: Findings of a 17-year prospective study of officially recorded and self-reported child abuse and neglect. *Child Abuse & Neglect, 22*(11), 1065–1078. http://dx.doi.org/10.1016/S0145-2134(98)00087-8.

Burke, M. M., Urbano, R. C., & Hodapp, R. M. (May 2011). Subsequent births in families of children with disabilities: Using demographic data to examine parents' reproductive patterns. *American Journal on Intellectual and Developmental Disabilities, 116*(3), 233–245. http://dx.doi.org/10.1352/1944-7558-116.3.233.

CDC. (2017). *Facts about ASDs*. Retrieved from http://www.cdc.gov/ncbddd/autism/facts.html.

Cheely, C. A., Carpenter, L. A., Letourneau, E. J., Nicholas, J. S., Charles, J., & King, L. B. (2012). The prevalence of youth with autism spectrum disorders in the criminal justice system. *Journal of Autism and Developmental Disorders, 42*(9), 1856–1862. http://dx.doi.org/10.1007/s10803-011-1427-2.

Christen, P. (2008). FEBRL: A freely available record linkage system with a graphical user interface. In *Proceedings of the second Australasian workshop on Health data and knowledge management* (Vol. 80) (pp. 17–25). Australian Computer Society, Inc.. Retrieved from http://dl.acm.org/citation.cfm?id=1385094.

Christensen, D. L. (2016). Prevalence and characteristics of autism spectrum disorder among children aged 8 years—Autism and Developmental Disabilities Monitoring Network, 11 Sites, United States, 2012. *MMWR. Surveillance Summaries, 65*. http://dx.doi.org/10.15585/mmwr.ss6503a1.

Crosse, S. B., Kaye, E., & Ratnofsky, A. (1992). *A report on the maltreatment of children with disabilities*. Arlington, VA: James Bell Associates, Inc. Retrieved from https://eric.ed.gov/?id=ED365089.

Department of Health and Human Services, Children's Bureau. (2014). *Differential response to reports of child abuse and neglect (child welfare information gateway)*. Washington, DC. Retrieved from https://www.childwelfare.gov/pubs/issue-briefs/differential-response/.

DiGiuseppe, D. L., Aron, D. C., Ranbom, L., Harper, D. L., & Rosenthal, G. E. (2002). Reliability of birth certificate data: A multi-hospital comparison to medical records information. *Maternal and Child Health Journal, 6*(3), 169–179. http://dx.doi.org/10.1023/A:1019726112597.

Duan, G., Chen, J., Zhang, W., Yu, B., Jin, Y., Wang, Y., & Yao, M. (2015). Physical maltreatment of children with autism in Henan province in China: A cross-sectional study. *Child Abuse & Neglect, 48*, 140–147. http://dx.doi.org/10.1016/j.chiabu.2015.03.018.

Elkins, T., del Aguinaga, M. P., Clinton-Selin, C., Clinton, B., & Gotterer, G. (2013). The maternal infant health outreach worker program in low-income families. *Journal of Health Care for the Poor and Underserved, 24*(3), 995–1001. http://dx.doi.org/10.1353/hpu.2013.0143.

Fisher, M. H., Hodapp, R. M., & Dykens, E. M. (2008). Child abuse among children with disabilities: What we know and what we need to know. In *B.-I. R. of R. in M. Retardation* (Vol. 35) (pp. 251–289). Academic Press. Retrieved from http://www.sciencedirect.com/science/article/pii/S0074775007350076.

Glaser, B. G. (1963). Retreading research materials: The use of secondary analysis by the independent researcher. *American Behavioral Scientist, 6*(10), 11–14. http://dx.doi.org/10.1177/000276426300601003.

Gomatam, S., Carter, R., Ariet, M., & Mitchell, G. (2002). An empirical comparison of record linkage procedures. *Statistics in Medicine, 21*(10), 1485–1496. http://dx.doi.org/10.1002/sim.1147.

Govindshenoy, M., & Spencer, N. (2007). Abuse of the disabled child: A systematic review of population-based studies. *Child: Care, Health and Development, 33*(5), 552–558. http://dx.doi.org/10.1111/j.1365-2214.2006.00693.x.

Hershkowitz, I., Lamb, M. E., & Horowitz, D. (2007). Victimization of children with disabilities. *American Journal of Orthopsychiatry*, 77(4), 629–635. http://dx.doi.org/10.1037/0002-9432.77.4.629.

Hexter, A. C., Harris, J. A., Roeper, P., Croen, L. A., Krueger, P., & Gant, D. (1990). Evaluation of the hospital discharge diagnoses index and the birth certificate as sources of information on birth defects. *Public Health Reports, 105*(3), 296.

Hodapp, R. M., Goldman, S. E., & Urbano, R. C. (2013). Using secondary datasets in disability research: Special issues, special promise. In *Using secondary datasets to understand persons with developmental disabilities and their families* (Vol. 45) (pp. 1–34).

Hodapp, R., Urbano, R., & So, S. (2006). Using an epidemiological approach to examine outcomes affecting young children with Down syndrome and their families. *Down Syndrome Research and Practice, 10*(2), 83–93.

Howlin, P., & Clements, J. (1995). Is it possible to assess the impact of abuse on children with pervasive developmental disorders? *Journal of Autism and Developmental Disorders, 25*(4), 337–354. http://dx.doi.org/10.1007/BF02179372.

Investigating Maltreatment. (July 4, 2017). Retrieved from https://www.tn.gov/dcs/article/investigating-maltreatment#sthash.WDJJKcby.dpuf.

Kirby, R. S. (2001). Invited commentary: Using vital statistics databases for perinatal epidemiology: Does the quality go in before the name goes on? *American Journal of Epidemiology, 154*(10), 889–890.

Lord, C., Rutter, M., DeLavore, P., Risi, S., Gotham, K., & Bishop, S. L. (2012). *Autism diagnostic observation schedule* (2nd ed.). Torrance, CA: Western Psychological Services (ADOS-2) Manual (Part I): Modules 1–4.
Mandell, D. S., Walrath, C. M., Manteuffel, B., Sgro, G., & Pinto-Martin, J. A. (2005). The prevalence and correlates of abuse among children with autism served in comprehensive community-based mental health settings. *Child Abuse & Neglect, 29*(12), 1359–1372. http://dx.doi.org/10.1016/j.chiabu.2005.06.006.
R Core Team. (2016). *R: A language and environment for statistical computing*. Vienna, Austria: R Foundation for Statistical Computing. Retrieved from https://www.R-project.org/.
Rutter, M., Le Couteur, A., & Lord, C. (2003). *Autism diagnostic interview-revised*. Los Angeles, CA: Western Psychological Services.
Sidebotham, P., & Heron, J. (May 15, 2006). Child maltreatment in the 'children of the nineties' : A cohort study of risk factors. *Child Abuse and Neglect, 30*(5), 497–522.
Spencer, N., Devereux, E., Wallace, A., Sundrum, R., Shenoy, M., Bacchus, C., & Logan, S. (September 2005). Disabling conditions and registration for child abuse and neglect: A population-based study. *Pediatrics, 116*(3), 609–613. http://dx.doi.org/10.1542/peds.2004-1882.
Spencer, N., Wallace, A., Sundrum, R., Bacchus, C., & Logan, S. (2006). Child abuse registration, fetal growth, and preterm birth: A population based study. *Journal of Epidemiology and Community Health, 60*(4), 337–340. http://dx.doi.org/10.1136/jech.2005.042085.
Sullivan, P. M., & Knutson, J. F. (2000). Maltreatment and disabilities: A population-based epidemiological study. *Child Abuse & Neglect, 24*(10), 1257–1273. http://dx.doi.org/10.1016/S0145-2134(00)00190-3.
Urbano, R. C., Beck, C., & Stephens, J. (2013). Linking datasets: A practical guide to research using secondary analysis. In *Using Secondary Datasets to Understand Persons with Developmental Disabilities and Their Families, 45* (pp. 35–121).
Urbano, R, C., & Hodapp, R. M. (2007). Divorce in families of children with down syndrome: A population-based study. *American Journal on Mental Retardation, 112*(4), 261–274.
Vizcarra, M., Cortés, J., Bustos, L., Alarcón, M. E, & Munoz, S. (December 2001). Child abuse in Temuco, Chile: Prevalence and risk factors. *Revista Médica de Chile, 129*(12), 1425–1432. http://dx.doi.org/10.4067/S0034-98872001001200008.
Wingate, M., Kirby, R. S., Pettygrove, S., Cunniff, C., Schulz, E., Ghosh, T., … Wright, V. (2014). Prevalence of autism spectrum disorder among children aged 8 years-autism and developmental disabilities monitoring network, 11 sites, United States, 2010. *MMWR Surveillance Summaries, 63*(2).
Wyckoff, A. S. (2011). AAP updates guidance on caring for children with Down syndrome. *AAP News*, 110725–110733. http://dx.doi.org/10.1542/aapnews.20110725-3.
Your Client's Rights. (July 4, 2017). Retrieved from https://www.tn.gov/dcs/topic/Your-Clients-Rights#sthash.9QiG4LyS.dpuf.

CHAPTER TWO

Peer Relationships Among Children With ASD: Interventions Targeting Social Acceptance, Friendships, and Peer Networks

Kyle Sterrett, Stephanie Shire, Connie Kasari[1]
University of California Los Angeles, Los Angeles, CA, United States
[1]Corresponding author: E-mail: kasari@gseis.ucla.edu

Contents

International Review of Research in Developmental Disabilities, Volume 52
ISSN 2211-6095
http://dx.doi.org/10.1016/bs.irrdd.2017.07.006

Abstract

Background: Developing meaningful friendships is an important protective factor for young children (Ladd, Kochenderfer, & Coleman, 1996; Rubin, LeMare, & Lollis, 1990) and is a skill with which children with autism spectrum disorder (ASD) often struggle (Chamberlain et al., 2007). Therefore, interventions targeting those skills play an important part in improving social outcomes.

Aim: The purpose of this review is to describe and examine the effectiveness of intervention trials that have targeted the development of friendship, peer networks, and discrete social skills (e.g., engagement, social initiations) in young children with ASD.

Method: Both single subject research designs (SSRDs) and randomized controlled trials (RCTs) examining interventions were evaluated for methodological quality (Logan, Hickman, Harris, & Heriza, 2008; Higgins & Green, 2011). Data regarding participant and study characteristics (i.e., age, gender, measures, intervention setting, approach, and effect sizes) were extracted from all included studies.

Results: 10 RCTs and 24 SSRDs with a combined sample size of 956 children were included. The majority of the interventions took place in children's schools and consistent effects were noted in increasing children's engagement with peers, especially when peer-mediated interventions (PMIs) were used. Less consistent effects were found for initiating, and responding to peers' social bids.

Discussion: PMIs appear to be a promising intervention approach to help children with ASD to engage with peers. Targeted interventions in general saw larger effects than comprehensive intervention packages. There was also a trend towards the implementation of interventions in natural contexts such as schools and the use of community members as the agent of intervention, improving the generalizability of the interventions. Understanding which approaches and intervention components work for specific targets remains an important direction for future research, there is also a clear need to evaluate critical outcomes such as friendship development, as friendship was rarely explicitly measured.

1. INTRODUCTION

Challenges and delays in the development of social communication skills are a core feature required for a diagnosis of autism spectrum disorder (ASD) (American Psychiatric Association, 2013). These delays can lead to marked differences between children with ASD and their typically developing peers (Palomo, Belinchón, & Ozonoff, 2006). Some differences noted for children with ASD include challenges sustaining social interactions with peers (Volkmar, Carter, Grossman, & Klin, 1997), initiating social bids (Hauck, Fein, Waterhouse, & Feinstein, 1995), and understanding the perspectives of others (Ozonoff & Miller, 1995).

Interventions have been developed to address these early delays in the development of social interaction and social communication skills, including joint attention (Kasari, Freeman, & Paparella, 2006), expressive language (Hardan et al., 2015), joint engagement (Kasari, Gulsrud, Paparella, Hellemann, & Berry, 2015), and shared attention with social partners (Green et al., 2010). Despite early intervention, delays often persist and can be exacerbated in school settings where peers are the expected social partners rather than supportive adults in therapeutic contexts. As such, difficulties in peer relationships, including social engagement and the development of friendships, can occur (Anderson, Locke, Kretzmann, Kasari, & Network, 2015; Rotheram-Fuller, Kasari, Chamberlain, & Locke, 2010). As school is where children spend a majority of their time, it is important to understand what can be done to improve the social outcomes of children with ASD in this setting.

To that end, it is also important to understand how research-based interventions are being implemented in school settings. This includes who is implementing the intervention, what skills are being targeted, how gains are measured, and what efforts are being made first to advance children's social outcomes and then to generalize and maintain those outcomes. Although gains have been demonstrated in clinic-based interventions on children's discrete social skills, such as social greetings and play skills with peers (Barry et al., 2003; Leaf et al., 2009), it is critical to examine how these interventions play out in school- and community-based real-world settings. A notable difference in community versus clinic implementation is the participation and training of community stakeholders, including school staff (Mandell et al., 2013; Stahmer et al., 2015). Community implementation of interventions within natural contexts, such as public schools, can increase equitable access to high-quality interventions. It is therefore important to evaluate the extent to which intervention studies have included community stakeholders and real-world environments through effectiveness trials and other design elements such as evaluating generalization of results.

The purpose of this review is to examine the intervention literature that has focused on improving the social experiences and friendships of preschool and elementary school age children with ASD. First, to evaluate which intervention approaches have the strongest evidence of efficacy and/or effectiveness specific to children's friendships/social connections or the theoretical prerequisite social skills to friendship such as social initiations and engagements with peers. Second, the methodological quality of research designs is examined to determine the level of confidence that can be placed in the conclusions drawn from the data. Third, the types of measures used to evaluate social constructs such as friendship and peer engagement are examined; measurement tools and the language used to describe the target outcomes vary widely in the literature. The measures used to evaluate change and the outcomes themselves will be discussed in the following sections.

2. REVIEW OF DESCRIPTIVE LITERATURE

Early observations by Kanner (1943) noted the social differences between children with ASD and their typically developing peers. In particular, he interpreted the behavior of children with ASD to be in a preferred state of "aloneness" stemming from a strong aversion to social stimuli. Central to Kanner's conception of children's desire for "aloneness" was the belief that poor social motivation resulted in a lack of friendships. In other words, he saw children with ASD as preferring to be alone with no social desire to develop friendships; social desire is necessary to feelings of loneliness, which is a negative appraisal of solitude or dissatisfaction with one's relationships (Margalit, 2012; Spitzberg & Hurt, 1987).

Although Kanner suggested that children with ASD lack social desire and that this lack of social desire leads to social isolation, contemporary research refutes this view. Studies have noted that children with ASD are often less skilled at friendship development and have difficulties initiating and maintaining social interactions (Sigman et al., 1999). It is a lack of skill (e.g., joint attention, language, functional play) and knowledge about others, not social desire that often prevents them from developing and sustaining positive relationships with their peers (Travis & Sigman, 1998). Moreover, when asked about feeling lonely at school, adolescents (but not children) are more likely to report loneliness than their neurotypical classmates (Bauminger & Kasari, 2000; Chamberlain et al., 2007). Thus, individuals with ASD have a social desire for friendships, as evident through feelings of loneliness, but seem to not have the knowledge or skills to achieve their friendship goals (Bauminger & Kasari, 2000; Bauminger, Shulman, & Agam, 2003).

2.1 Experience and Context

Children with ASD have difficulties with early social communication and social connectivity (Adamson, Bakeman, Deckner, & Romski, 2009; Dawson et al., 2004). However, the extent to which these early delays are exacerbated by contextual factors such as the amount and quality of social opportunities presented to children is less clear. Friendships develop from contact and positive experiences with others. Because children with ASD often have fewer experiences with their peers, they are at a disadvantage for learning about and interacting with others, thus developing successful friendships. There may be several reasons why children have fewer peer experiences, including taxing therapy schedules involving one-on-one sessions with adults, segregated schooling contexts that resemble more adult–child therapy contexts, and self-isolation in group contexts so that peer interactions are limited. One common goal for many families is to place their children with ASD (often verbal children) within inclusive classrooms.

Although inclusion is often viewed as the best context to help children with ASD hone their social skills and develop friendships, the data are mixed. Several studies of classroom social networks indicate that children with ASD fully included in general education classrooms are more involved in their class peer interactions than Kanner (1943) would have predicted. Two studies demonstrate that few children are identified as isolated in classroom social network surveys, and some are even popular, meaning they have many social connections within the class (Chamberlain et al., 2007; Kasari, Locke, Gulsrud, & Rotheram-Fuller, 2011). It is less well understood how these connections continue throughout the school year. Over time, social networks including children with ASD can become *fragmented*, meaning that children who nominated each other as friends early in the year did not always make those same nominations again at the end of the year (Anderson et al., 2015; Rotheram-Fuller et al., 2010). This suggests that it is difficult for children with ASD to maintain the friendships that they do make. Despite this variability over time, similarly to their typically developing peers, elementary age children with ASD also report very low levels of loneliness (Chamberlain et al., 2007). However, preadolescents and adolescents in inclusive settings report more loneliness at school, and they generally report poorer quality friendships compared with their neurotypical classmates (Bauminger & Kasari, 2000).

2.2 Role of Gender

Studies with elementary school children with ASD indicate differences in friendships for boys and girls. For example, boys have greater social connectivity to their classmates in smaller classrooms during the early grades in elementary school, whereas girls do better in larger classrooms at the older, fourth and fifth, grade levels (Anderson et al., 2015; Locke, Kasari, Rotheram-Fuller, Kretzmann, & Jacobs, 2013). Recent work also highlights potential differences in girls' playground behavior. For example, girls have been found to use compensatory strategies to "camouflage" social difficulties such as staying near to peers and superficially joining into group activities (i.e., present within the group but not jointly engaged). The structured nature of predominately male activities (e.g., handball, kickball) does not allow for that sort of fleeting engagement and so boys are more visibly isolated when not a part of those games (Dean et al., 2014; Dean, Harwood, & Kasari, 2016). Therefore, gender may be an important factor to consider when planning social interventions at school.

2.3 The Importance of Intervention

In the neurotypical literature, for young students there is a relationship between close friendships early on in the school year and improved attitudes and positive feelings toward school (Ladd et al., 1996). The converse is also true, where students with high levels of conflict with peers show less engagement in and enjoyment of school. Additionally, social isolation, defined here as the lack of close friendships, has been linked to negative self-esteem and self-worth in children (Rubin et al., 1990). However, having friends serves as a protective factor against these potentially negative outcomes (Parker, Saxon, Asher, & Kovacs, 1999). Friendships can provide clear benefits and protection from negative outcomes including protection against harm that may come directly from bullying or victimization (Hodges, Boivin, Vitaro, & Bukowski, 1999). Considering the challenges specific to peer interactions faced by young children with ASD, interventions targeting friendships and social acceptance represent an important target.

For children with ASD, early social delays may influence the amount and quality of social opportunities presented and these experiences, in turn, may also influence their social growth. As such, interventions targeting both social skills and the children's social environment's (such as the quality of social opportunities provided to children) are necessary to improve children's outcomes. These interventions must take into account factors such as gender in order to improve the chances of success but have the potential to affect a number of critical outcomes such as self-esteem and positive feelings towards school. The purpose of this review is to determine what steps can be taken to address those outcomes. This will be done through an evaluation of intervention effects, the tools used to measure those effects, and the methodological quality of the trials where those interventions have been tested.

3. METHOD

3.1 Search Strategy

In December of 2016, a full search of five electronic databases (ProQuest, ERIC, Web of Science, MEDLINE/PubMed, and Google Scholar) was carried out. Search terms focused on children with ASD, behavioral interventions, and social outcomes including friendship and social acceptance. The search was limited to articles written in English and Grey literature (e.g., dissertations and unpublished theses) was excluded. No restrictions were placed on the date of publication. A full description of the exact search strings used for each database is provided in Table 1.

3.2 Study Selection

Included studies met the following criteria:

1. Used an experimental design, either a single subject research design (SSRD) or a randomized controlled trial (RCT). This excludes all quasiexperimental or preexperimental designs (e.g., AB designs, pre-post no control).
2. Included children with a diagnosis of autism or related disorders (e.g., Asperger's or pervasive developmental disorder—not otherwise specified). Diagnostic information could be provided by the study team [e.g., administration of the Autism Diagnostic Observation Schedule (ADOS, Lord et al., 2012) or Autism Diagnostic Interview-Revised (ADI-R, Le Couteur, Lord, & Rutter, 2003)] or through review of records including a clinical diagnosis from outside the study team (e.g., reference to DSM criterion) or review of school records.

Table 1 Search Strings for Online Databases

	Search String
ProQuest	ab(Pervasive develop OR Autis[a] OR Asperger[a]) AND ab(school age[a] OR Primary School OR elementary[a] OR pre-school OR K-2 OR 3-5) AND ab(Friend[a] OR Social acceptance OR peer relation[a] OR peer networks OR social networks OR social relationship OR friendship quality OR isolation OR rejection OR social adjustment OR victim[a] OR bull[a] OR exclusion) AND ab(Intervention OR Program OR Group OR Train[a] OR Social skills training OR teacher OR parent OR peer mediated)
ERIC	("Pervasive developmental Disorder" OR Autism OR ASD OR Asperger) AND ("school age" OR "Primary School" OR elementary OR pre-school OR K-2 OR 3-5) AND (Friend OR "Social acceptance" OR "peer relationships" OR "peer networks" OR "social networks" OR "social relationship" OR "friendship quality" OR isolation OR rejection OR "social adjustment" OR victim OR bully OR exclusion) AND (intervention OR Program OR Group OR training OR "Social skills training" OR teacher OR parent OR "peer mediated")
Web of Science	(TS = (("Pervasive developmental Disorder" OR Autism OR ASD OR Asperger) AND ("school age" OR "Primary School" OR elementary OR pre-school OR K-2 OR 3-5) AND (Friend OR "Social acceptance" OR "peer relationships" OR "peer networks" OR "social networks" OR "social relationship" OR "friendship quality" OR isolation OR rejection OR "social adjustment" OR victim OR bully OR exclusion) AND (Intervention OR Program OR Group OR Training OR "Social skills training" OR teacher OR parent OR "peer mediated"))) *AND* **LANGUAGE**:(English) **Timespan**: All years. **Indexes**: SCI-EXPANDED, SSCI, A&HCI, CPCI-S, CPCI-SSH, BKCI-S, BKCI-SSH, ESCI, CCR-EXPANDED, IC.
PubMed	((((Pervasive develop[a] OR Autis[a] OR Asperger[a])) AND (school age[a] OR Primary School OR elementary[a] OR pre-school OR K-2 OR 3-5)) AND (Friend[a] OR Social acceptance OR peer relation[a] OR peer networks OR social networks OR social relationship OR friendship quality OR isolation OR rejection OR social adjustment OR victim[a] OR bully[a] OR exclusion)) AND (Intervention OR Program OR Group OR Train[a] OR Social skills training OR teacher OR parent OR peer mediated)

Table 1 Search Strings for Online Databases—cont'd

	Search String
Google Scholar[a]	("Pervasive developmental Disorder" OR Autism OR ASD OR Asperger) AND ("school age" OR "Primary School" OR elementary OR pre-school OR K-2 OR 3-5) AND (Friend OR "Social acceptance" OR "peer relationships" OR "peer networks" OR "social networks" OR "social relationship" OR "friendship quality" OR isolation OR rejection OR "social adjustment" OR victim OR bully OR exclusion) AND (Intervention OR Program OR Group OR Training OR "Social skills training" OR teacher OR parent OR "peer mediated")

[a]Stopped at page 23 as searches were no longer relevant.

3. The mean age of the participants fell within 4–11 years of age (preschool and elementary school age children).
4. The primary dependent variable focused on friendship and social acceptance or the converse, social rejection, and bullying. Discrete social skills such as initiating and responding to communication bids with peers were also included as they are often considered foundational to friendship development.
5. Published in a peer-reviewed journal in the English language.

3.3 Ratings of Methodological Quality

Two measures of methodological quality were needed to separately address SSRDs and RCTs. To evaluate the studies using SSRDs, a subsection focusing on research design of a published rating scale of methodological quality was used (Logan et al., 2008). The three-item subscale evaluates experimental control and the research design, namely (1) Was the type of SSRD clearly and correctly stated? (2) Were there an adequate number of data points in each phase (at least 5)? and (3) Were the effects of the intervention replicated across three or more subjects? These were each answered on a binary, yes or no, scale. The studies were deemed as having sound methodology and design only when each of the three criteria was met. A random 20% of the SSRD studies were double coded by independent raters and there was 100% agreement between coders on ratings of methodological quality.

For the RCTs a subset of the questions from the Cochrane review standards for methodological quality was used (Higgins & Green, 2011). These criteria have been used in similar reviews in autism-related research (e.g., Oono, Honey, & McConachie, 2013). A subset of five of the seven criteria were used for the purpose of this review of behavioral interventions: (1) Were randomization procedures clearly stated and properly used? (2) Was randomization successful in producing similar groups at baseline? (3) Were assessors blind to group status? (4) Were there incomplete data as a result of missing data or attrition? (5) Were there clearly stated primary and secondary outcomes? (Lack of prespecified outcomes may increase the risk for reporting bias such as reporting spuriously significant results and nonreporting of nonsignificant results.) Two items specific to medical trials were excluded, the blinding of participants and the concealing of the randomization. Three options were available in producing these ratings, yes, no, and unclear. Meeting these five criteria improves confidence in the internal validity of the intervention trial. Thirty percent of studies were double coded by two independent raters (ICC = 0.923).

3.4 Intervention Effects

The effects of the SSRD were evaluated using the percentage of nonoverlapping data (PND) metric, which calculates the number of data points in the intervention phase that are greater than the most extreme baseline data points (Lenz, 2013). The rule of thumb for interpreting these data are as follows: 0–50% of nonoverlapping data show an intervention is noneffective, 50–69% show debatable effectiveness, 70–89% indicate moderate effectiveness, and 90–100% indicate an effective intervention (Scruggs & Mastropieri, 1998).

For RCTs, statistical significance (e.g., *p*-values) is a common metric used to determine the success of an intervention trial. However, statistical significance is confounded by sample size and so these results should be interpreted with caution. When possible, measures of effect size were used and consisted primarily of standardizing the mean differences (e.g., Cohen's d). If a measure such as Cohen's d was not provided, statistical significance was used as the metric for efficacy.

3.5 Data Extraction

Data extracted across all studies included age of the participants, sample size, gender, intervention context (e.g., school, home clinic), intervention approach (e.g., direct instruction, peer-mediated), intervention provider, measurement of maintenance and generalization, and effect size (RCTs).

4. RESULTS

4.1 Search Results

The total number of articles that were produced by the searches of the five electronic databases was 873. Google Scholar produced many more results; however, the search was halted after 220 articles due to the lack of overlap between the articles and search criteria (long string of irrelevant articles). Of the 873 articles, 69 abstracts were selected for review, based on their relevance to the search terms and research questions, and were subjected to examination for the full inclusion criteria. From those, 17 were classified as descriptive studies and so were not included in the primary analyses. The 34 studies that met full inclusion criteria consist of 24 SSRDs and 10 RCTs. A quorum diagram is provided (Fig. 1).

4.2 Methodological Quality Ratings

4.2.1 Single Subject Research Designs

The majority of the included studies utilized SSRDs. The 24 SSRD studies included 20 multiple baseline designs, 3 reversal designs (Gonzalez-Lopez & Kamps, 1997; Koegel, Werner, Vismara, & Koegel, 2005; Laushey & Heflin, 2000), and 1 alternating treatment design (Wilson, 2013). Each of

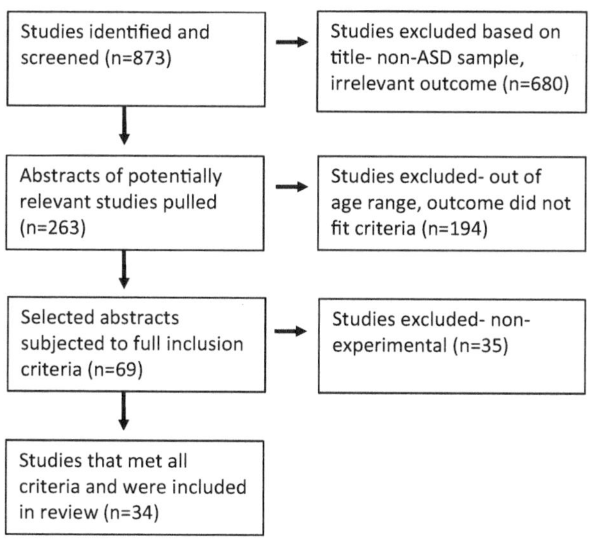

Figure 1 Quorum diagram of study inclusion process.

the studies was rated in terms of the quality of their designs based on the criteria established by Logan et al. (2008). Only three studies met each of those criteria (Hartzell, Liaupsin, Gann, & Clem, 2015; Mason et al., 2014; Thiemann & Goldstein, 2004). Nearly half of the studies failed to demonstrate three replications of experimental control (n = 12), while nine studies had less than five data points within phases. See Table 2.

Ten studies measured maintenance of the skills that were targeted by the intervention and nine measured the generalization of the skills in a different context than the target was taught. Of those, four studies measured both maintenance as well as generalization (Feldman & Matos, 2013; Hartzell et al., 2015; Koegel, Kuriakose, Singh, & Koegel, 2012; Laushey, Heflin, Shippen, Alberto, & Fredrick, 2009).

4.2.2 Randomized Controlled Trials

A summary of methodological ratings for the RCTs is provided in Table 3. None of the included studies met all the criteria. Two studies had nonspecified randomization procedures (Roeyers, 1996; Wood, Fujii, Renno, & Van Dyke, 2014) and three did not have blinded assessors (Frankel et al., 2010; Kamps et al., 2015; Roeyers, 1996). Other frequently identified design challenges included missing outcome data due to attrition (n = 6), a lack of in-text description of prespecified primary and secondary outcomes (n = 6), and a lack of description of statistical verification of group similarities at baseline (n = 3). Consistent efforts were made to measure maintenance and generalization in the RCTs. Six studies included a follow-up period to measure the maintenance of the targeted skills and seven included a measure of generalization.

4.3 Participant and Intervention Characteristics

4.3.1 Single Subject Research Designs

There were a total of 77 target children with ASD enrolled in kindergarten through sixth grade classrooms who were included across the SSRD studies. In addition, peer models were included in 11 studies. In terms of confirming diagnoses, only one study used a research assessment (i.e., ADOS and ADI-R). Of the others, the most common method was reliance on a diagnostic evaluation from an external agency or psychologist (n = 17), other methods included review of educational records (n = 5) or parental reports (n = 1); two studies did not specify how a

Table 2 Overview of Extracted Information From Single Subject Research Designs

	Sample Size (Female)	Age Range	Follow-Up	Generalization	Intervention Approach	Context	Outcome	Effects	Meets All Three Methodological Standards
Banda et al. (2010)	2(0)	6	No	No	Peer/direct instruction	School	Frequency count: initiations and responses	Initiations: 100% Responses: 100%	No
Barber et al. (2016)	3(0)	3–4	Yes	No	Peer	Clinic	Frequency count: initiations and responses	Initiations: 17% Responses: 85%	No
Brady et al. (1987)	2(2)	8–10	Yes	No	Peer	School	Interval coding: initiations	Initiations to trained peers: 52%	No
Feldman and Matos (2013)	3(0)	5–8	Yes	Yes	Direct instruction	School	Interval coding: reciprocal social interactions	Reciprocal interactions: 93%	No
Gena (2006)	4(2)	4	No	Yes	Direct instruction	School	Frequency count: initiations and responses	Initiations 95% Responses 98%	No
Gonzalez-Lopez and Kamps (1997)	4(2)	5–7	No	No	Peer	School	Frequency count: interactions	Peer interactions: 54%	No
Harper et al. (2008)	2(0)	8–9	No	Yes	Peer	School	Frequency count: gaining attention, initiations, turn-taking	Gaining Attention: 94% Initiations: 16% Turn-taking: 100%	No
Hartzell et al. (2015)	3(3)	6	Yes	Yes	Direct instruction	School	Time sampling: time in engagement	Engagement 100%	Yes
Kamps et al. (2014)	4(1)	6–7	No	Yes	Direct instruction	School	Frequency count: total communication initiations and responses	Total communication: 86% Initiations: 45% Responses: 73%	No
Koegel et al. (2005)	2(1)	8–9	No	No	Direct instruction	Community	Interval coding: synchronous interaction with peer	Synchronous interactions: 100%	No

(*Continued*)

Table 2 Overview of Extracted Information From Single Subject Research Designs—cont'd

	Sample Size (Female)	Age Range	Follow-Up	Generalization	Intervention Approach	Context	Outcome	Effects	Meets All Three Methodological Standards
Koegel, Kuriakose, et al. (2012)	3(1)	5–6	Yes	Yes	Direct instruction	School	Frequency count/time in engagement: initiations; social engagement; affect	Engagement: 80% Initiations: 40% Affect 83%	No
Koegel, Vernon, Koegel, Koegel, & Paullin (2012)	3(1)	9–12	No	No	Direct instruction	School	Time in engagement/ frequency count	Engagement: 95% Initiations 95%	No
Koegel et al. (2014)	3(1)	5–9	Yes	No	Direct instruction	School	Interval coding: engagement with peers. Frequency count: initiations	Engagement: 100% Initiations: 94%	No
Laushey and Heflin (2000)	2(0)	5	No	No	Peer	School	Percent of successful opportunities: requesting; gaining attention; waiting turn; orienting toward social partner	Social skills: 100%	No
Laushey et al. (2009)	4(0)	6–9	Yes	Yes	Peer/direct instruction	School	Proportion correct: responses, initiations, recognition of nonverbal cues	Responses: 91% Initiations: 100% Recognition of facial expressions: 100%	No
Leaf et al. (2009)	3(0)	5–7	Yes	No	Direct instruction	Clinic	Partial time interval: play skills, frequency of conversation within intervals. Positive emotions	Play: 85% Conversation: 89% Emotion 100%	No

Mason et al. (2014)	3(0)	6–8	No	No	Peer/direct instruction	School	Frequency count: total number of communicative acts	Communicative acts: 97%	Yes
Mundschenk and Sasso (1995)	3(1)	7–9	No	No	Peer	School	Partial interval coding: responses, sustained interactions	Responses: 37% Sustained interactions: 25%	No
Owen-DeSchryver et al. (2008)	3(0)	7–10	No	Yes	Peer	School	Interval coding: initiations and responses	Initiations: 59% Responses: 63%	No
Radley et al. (2014)	4(0)	8–10	No	No	Direct instruction	School	Frequency count: initiations and responses and proportion of time engaged	Engagement: 77% Initiations: 55% Responses: 58%	No
Rosenberg et al. (2015)	3(1)	6–7	No	No	Direct instruction	School	Frequency of social exchanges	Social exchanges: 100%	No
Shafer et al. (1984)	4(1)	5–6	No	Yes	Peer	School	Interval coding: prosocial behaviors directed toward peer	Prosocial behavior: 74%	No
Thiemann and Goldstein (2004)	5(0)	6–9	Yes	No	Direct instruction	School	Frequency of six prosocial behaviors	Prosocial behaviors: 51%	Yes
Wilson (2013)	4(2)	3–5	Yes	No	Direct instruction	School	Frequency count: nonverbal communication	Reach: in vivo (IV): 60%, video modeling (VM): 40%. Gesture to request IV: 29%, VM: 57%. Pointing/vocalization IV: 0%, VM: 0%	No

Effects calculated using the percentage of nonoverlapping data. Methodological standards rating is based on meeting all three criteria from the research design and experimental control subscales established by Logan et al. (2008).

Table 3 Methodological Quality Ratings for Randomized Controlled Trials

	Random Sequence Generation	Successful Randomization	Blinded Outcome Assessor	Incomplete Outcome Data	Specified A Priori Outcomes
Frankel et al. (2010)	Yes	Yes	No	Yes	No
Kamps et al. (2015)	Yes	Unclear	No	Yes	Yes
Kasari et al. (2012)	Yes	No[a]	Yes	No	Yes
Kasari et al. (2016)	Yes	No[a]	Yes	Yes[b]	Yes
Koning et al. (2013)	Yes	Yes	Yes	No	No
Kretzmann et al. (2015)	Yes	Yes	Yes	No	Yes
Roeyers (1996)	Unclear	Yes	Unclear	Unclear	No
Soorya et al. (2015)	Yes	Yes	Yes	Yes[b]	No
Wood et al. (2014)	Unclear	Yes	Yes	No	No
Young et al. (2016)	Yes	Yes[a]	Yes	Yes[b]	No

[a]Differences present but controlled for in analysis.
[b]Attrition at follow-up but not at exit of the study.

diagnosis was made (studies sometimes used multiple methods such as external evaluation and a review of educational records).

The majority of participants were male (n = 58, 75%). The children included in these studies tended to be verbal and were able to participate in mainstream educational settings. Students who needed additional support were not represented. Information was not provided as to whether the children met clinical criteria for comorbid diagnoses such as anxiety; however, studies often included stipulations in the inclusion criteria such as having a lack of disruptive behaviors.

Most (n = 22) of the intervention trials took place in the context of children's schools and were conducted during recess, in classrooms, and in separate rooms within the school. Only two trials took place outside of schools, with one in a clinic setting and one in the child's home and community (e.g., park or local zoo).

4.3.2 Randomized Controlled Trials

There were a total of 879 children across the 10 included studies with sample sizes ranging from 13 to 302 participants (median = 68 participants). These numbers include only the children with ASD, who were the targets of intervention, and not peer models, aides, or other staff. Of the 879 children, only 20% were female, although this discrepancy is expected due to the differential rate of diagnosis across genders. The mean age was approximately 8— years old. Nearly all participants were verbal and had an IQ greater than 70. Only one RCT explicitly included children with cognitive impairments (Roeyers, 1996). Inclusion criteria relating to IQ and verbal abilities were assessed using a variety of measures including parent and teacher reports and norm-referenced measures (e.g., Kaufman Brief Intelligence Test, Second Edition and Stanford Binet-5). One hundred and thirty-five school staff were recruited and trained to implement interventions across three RCTs (Kamps et al., 2015; Kretzmann, Shih, & Kasari, 2015; Young, Falco, & Hanita, 2016). These staff included playground aides, teachers, speech language pathologists, and resource room teachers. Demographic information for participating adults was collected in only a few studies. When reported, staff were predominately female (Kretzmann et al., 2015), had taught for an average of about 15 years, and had earned Master's degrees (Young et al., 2016).

In terms of the settings of the RCTs, six of the interventions took place in children's schools and the other four in clinic settings. Only one of the interventions utilized a peer-mediated approach (compared to a business as usual control), eight utilized direct instruction, and one study compared direct instruction to a peer-mediated approach. Of those studies which took a direct instruction approach, four were provided by trained clinicians and four were provided by parents, teachers, or paraprofessionals with clinician support. Lastly, looking further at the measurement of the targeted skills in the intervention trials, six of the studies measured maintenance of the target skills and seven measured generalization to natural social contexts; only three of the 10 measured both.

4.4 Intervention Protocols

4.4.1 Single Subject Research Designs

A wide range of intervention approaches were utilized across the included studies. The use of the principles of Pivotal Response Treatment (PRT) was common in the SSRD interventions (n = 5). These interventions relied on strategies such as varying the activities used to teach, narrating play, gaining attention, reinforcing social attempts, turn-taking, and using motivating activities and materials (Harper, Symon, & Frea, 2008). Motivating activities and reinforcing appropriate social attempts were common strategies used to increase the probability that the target skills, such as initiating to peers, would occur. PRT strategies were used in a number of ways. The sessions were set up with the environment designed to be socially enticing, such as creating a "lunch club" with peers based on the child's interests (e.g., Koegel, Vernon, et al., 2012), explicitly teaching peers to execute PRT strategies when interacting with children with ASD (Harper et al., 2008), direct use of PRT by an adult (Feldman & Matos, 2013), or teaching aides to implement the strategies (Koegel, Kim & Koegel, 2014).

In peer-mediated interventions (n = 11), peers were didactically taught skills including being patient and waiting for social initiations, how to invite friends to join games, and asking questions. Beyond these didactic lessons, strategies such as guided practice of the skills through prompting (Banda, Hart, & Liu-Gitz, 2010), retrospective review of past play with target children (Kamps et al., 2014), and reinforcement of successful attempts to include target children (Mason et al., 2014) were used to teach peer models.

Across the remaining studies, the use of video modeling (watching a video of the target skill being performed correctly: Wilson, 2013), social scripts (Gonzalez-Lopez & Kamps, 1997), and visual prompts with pictures followed by reinforcement (Rosenberg, Congdon, Schwartz, & Kamps, 2015) were among the strategies used in the interventions.

4.4.2 Randomized Controlled Trials

The peer-mediated interventions tested using RCTs (Kasari, Rotheram-Fuller, Locke, & Gulsrud, 2012; Roeyers, 1996) utilized the same intervention principles as the SSRDs such as didactic lessons with the peer models and providing guided practice. Methods of direct instruction varied; however, one approach in particular, cognitive behavior therapy (CBT), was tested in two of the RCTs but none of the SSRDs (Koning, Magill-Evans, Volden, & Dick, 2013; Wood et al., 2014). CBT is a multicomponent intervention that simultaneously targets multiple behaviors, such as social anxiety, through guided exposure, social coaching through the lens of understanding the thoughts and feelings of peers, practice of skills, such as being a good friend and entering games in live situations, and lastly the reinforcement of correctly utilizing intervention strategies (Wood et al., 2014).

The training of playground aides was used as the method of intervention to target children's social skills and peer connections in two SSRDs (Feldman & Matos, 2013; Koegel et al., 2014) and one RCT (Kretzmann et al., 2015). The training protocol for the RCT consisted of active in vivo coaching of the aides and the systematic fading of the coaching and support. The strategies taught to the aides included monitoring children's engagement, starting a structured game or activity on the playground, and facilitating inclusion and social success for children within the games and activities (Kretzmann et al., 2015). Other strategies that were taught include incorporating children's preferred interests and maintaining an appropriate distance from the child (Koegel et al., 2014).

The final study incorporated a "comprehensive treatment model" where children with ASD were taught throughout the day using environmental and visual supports as well as using incidental teaching strategies across both social and nonsocial routines to teach appropriate social skills (Young et al., 2016). Through this model, children are provided with many opportunities to learn and practice appropriate social skills and develop peer relationships throughout the school day as the teacher facilitates interactions between peers. Additionally, individual didactic lessons are incorporated to build requisite social skills through more personalized instruction.

4.5 Intervention Targets and Outcome Measures

Across the included studies there were a number of commonly utilized measures describing friendship, social skills, and social acceptance in ASD. These measures assessed a range of different reporters including student self-reports, parents, teachers, and direct observations by trained clinicians. Careful consideration of the strengths and potential bias of each type of measure is needed when evaluating outcomes based on the different methods.

4.5.1 Self-Report: Social Networks and Friendships

The evaluation of children's social networks and friendships through self-report is a relatively new measurement technique that offers a unique perspective into the overall classroom social environment. Self-report surveys such as the Social Network Survey (also known as Friendship Survey) have been used to provide a stable picture of children's friendships within inclusive and special education classrooms (Cairns, Cairns, Neckerman, Gest, & Gariepy, 1988).

The procedure for this survey is simple and involves asking all of the children in the class questions such as, "Are there any kids in your class who like to hang out together?" The responses are recorded and from these responses a list of different social groups (social connections) and the position of specific children within those groups (social centrality) can be generated. For example, a child could be central to a group including two other children but that group may not share many other connections within the class and therefore the child will be considered to be at the periphery of the classroom social structure.

Self-reported friendships can be measured using the same survey with additional questions asking for children to nominate friends within their class. These questions produce a frequency count of the number of friends that children nominate within their class, the number of close friends that they nominate, the reciprocity of those friendships (whether children nominated each other), and lastly produces a frequency count of those children whose peers do not like to socialize with them. The Social Network/Friendship survey was used as an outcome in two of the RCTs (Kasari et al., 2012; Kasari et al., 2016).

One limitation of self-report measures is the difficulty of administration. They are typically more time intensive and rely heavily on recall, which may be difficult for some children with ASD. Additionally, in administering this measure to younger children (kindergarten and first grade) who cannot yet write, researchers must administer the measures in small groups or one-to-one settings, and the children may require more prompting or explanation of the questions to produce appropriate responses, contributing both to the cost of administration and potentially biasing results if assessors inadvertently lead children to nominate some classmates over others.

4.5.2 Parent and Teacher Report: Social Network and Friendships

Measures such as the Friendship Qualities Scale (Bukowski, Hoza & Bolvin, 1994) are efficient data collection tools and provide access to caregivers' perceptions of children's peer relationships. Other measures such as the Teacher Impression Scale (Odom et al., 1997) provide data on children's social skills from the perspective of the educational staff. The Social Responsiveness Scale (SRS—Constantino et al., 2003) is a measure of ASD symptomatology and can be completed by both teachers and caregivers. In addition, norm-referenced parent report measures such as the Vineland Adaptive Behaviors Scale (used in three RCTs: Kamps et al., 2015; Koning et al., 2013; Young et al., 2016) are used to provide a more holistic view of children's broad social functioning. Although frequently applied, these types of measures have a number of limitations. For example, reports from external observers do not capture the reciprocity of the friendships directly and may vary depending on the context that the reporter sees the child interact with peers. Parent and teacher report measures were not used as an outcome in any SSRD study but were used in five of the 10 RCTs. Teacher reports were used less frequently, only three times.

4.5.3 Direct Observation: Peer Engagement

Direct observational measures of engagement were the most common type of assessment used in SSRD studies appearing in over half (see Table 2) and were also used in six of the ten RCTs (see Table 4). Direct observations consist of an assessor watching the child and live coding (e.g., interval measurements or frequency counts) for the target behavior in natural or seminatural social interactions with peers or adults. Definitions of the social outcome referred to as "engagement" varied across studies. For example, Koegel, Vernon, Koegel, Koegel, and Paullin (2012) defined engagement as remaining in the same area as the peers and interacting with them, while Hartzell et al. (2015) included a more comprehensive definition including appropriate body language, eye contact, and audibility of speech. Kasari and Rotheram-Fuller (2005) defined joint engagement as directed social behavior between a child and peer within a turn-taking structure. Therefore, the term "engagement" encompasses a wide range of behaviors from a lenient standard of being in physical proximity to peers through to the quality of the child's social behavior in interactions with peers. It is important to be cognizant of the way that constructs are defined across the studies to understand what behaviors are being influenced by the intervention and what are not. For example, studies with more stringent definitions of engagement that required sustained interactions (multiple back and forth social turns) saw smaller effects (Gonzalez-Lopez & Kamps, 1997; Mundschenk & Sasso, 1995) compared with studies that merely required directed communication or responses to social bids to constitute engagement (Hartzell et al., 2015). Looking at the RCTs, large effects on engagement were seen despite a more stringent definition (e.g., Kretzmann et al., 2015).

Table 4 Overview of Extracted Information From Randomized Controlled Trials

	Sample Size	Percent Female (%)	Mean Age	Follow-up	Generalization	Intervention Approach	Context	Provider	Outcome Measure	Statistically Significant Effects[a]
Frankel et al. (2010)	68	15	8.5	Yes	No	Direct instruction	Clinic	Clinician/ parent	Loneliness scale; QPQ; SSRS; PEI; PHS	Loneliness, popularity, assertion, and self-control[b]
Kamps et al. (2015)	95	16	5.8	No	Yes	Direct instruction	School	Teacher	CELF; VABS; TIS; direct observation	CELF; VABS-communication; initiations, and communication[b]
Kasari et al. (2012)	60	10	8.2	Yes	Yes	Both	School	Clinician/ peer	Friendship survey; POPE	Peer mediated: social network salience d = 0.79; time solitary d = 0.94
Kasari et al. (2016)	148	26	8.2	Yes	Yes	Direct instruction	School	Clinician	Friendship survey; POPE; STRS	SNS moderated by STRS; skills: joint engagement[b]
Koning et al. (2013)	15	0	11.1	No	Yes	Direct instruction	Clinic	Clinician	VABS; SRS; ADOS; direct observation; knowledge test	Peer interactions d = 0.29; CASP d = 0.45–0.61; social knowledge d = 0.68
Kretzmann et al. (2015)	24	25	7.5	Yes	Yes	Direct instruction	School	Classroom aide	POPE	Engagement d = 1.27
Roeyers (1996)	85	33	9.3	No	Yes	Peer mediated	School	Peer	Direct observation	Engagement; responses and initiations[b]

Soorya et al. (2015)	69	17	9.9	Yes	No	Direct instruction	Clinic	Clinician	SRS; GEM; CCC; DANVA; SST; RMET	Positive social behaviors d = 0.88[c]
Wood et al. (2014)	13	23	8.8	No	Yes	Direct instruction	Clinic	Clinician	POPE	Time solitary d = 1.47; time in peer interactions d = 1.36; positive interactions d = 1.62; responses d = 1.34; negative behavior d = 0.5
Young et al. (2016)	302	20	4.4	Yes	No	Direct instruction	School	Teacher	CARS; VABS; BDI; EOWPVT; ROWPVT; ASIEP; SSRS	Receptive language g = 0.13; SSRS g = 0.19

ADOS, autism diagnostic observation schedule; *ASIEP*, autism screening instrument for educational planning; *BDI*, battelle developmental inventory; *CARS*, child autism rating scale; *CCC*, child communication checklist; *CELF*, clinical evaluation of language fundamentals; *DANVA*, diagnostic analysis of nonverbal accuracy; *EOWPVT*, expressive one-word picture vocabulary test; *GEM*, Griffith empathy measure; *PEI*, the pupil evaluation inventory; *PHSCS*, Piers—Harris self-concept scale; *POPE*, playground observation of peer engagement; *QPP*, quality of play questionnaire; *RMET*, reading the mind in the eyes task; *ROWPVT*, receptive one-word picture vocabulary test; *SNS*, social network salience; *SRS*, social responsiveness scale; *SSRS*, social skills rating system; *SST*, strange stories task; *STRS*, student teacher relationship scale; *TIS*, teacher impression scale; *VABS*, Vineland adaptive behavior scale.

[a]Nonsignificant results are not included in the table.

[b]Statistically significant but no effect size reported.

[c]Effects not maintained at follow-up.

One specific observational measure, the Playground Observation of Peer Engagement (POPE – Kasari and Rotheram-Fuller, 2005), was used in four RCT studies (Kasari et al., 2016, 2012; Kretzmann et al., 2015; Wood et al., 2014). The POPE is a 10-min observation that takes place during children's free time at school (e.g., recess and lunch) where mutually exclusive engagement states are identified on 1-min intervals from solitary (physically distant and/or not engaged in play or socialization with another peer) through to jointly engaged (e.g., reading a comic together or engaged in reciprocal conversation). Joint engagement refers to a state (period of time) where the child notices another peer and coordinates their attention between the peer and a shared activity. Therefore, for a child to be considered "jointly engaged," this requires more than just proximity and awareness of the social partner, what is required is active social connectivity. Joint engagement can be paired with verbal initiations and responses or not. For example, two children who are playing catch together without talking can be jointly engaged, and two children discussing and pointing out pictures in a favorite comic book can also be considered jointly engaged.

The remaining two studies utilized various observational methods including video recordings of natural peer interactions coded for engagement with peers (Roeyers, 1996) and video recordings of contrived interactions with a confederate, coded for both verbal and nonverbal engagement. The definition Roeyers (1996) provided for engagement is different from the POPE. Intervals in which the children initiate or respond to peers are considered to be intervals of engagement.

4.5.4 Direct Observation: Initiations and Responses

Children's social initiations and responses to social bids are a common target of intervention and are viewed as requisite skills to develop friendships. Studies measure this construct in a number of different contexts including in classrooms, contrived or manipulated social situations, and on the playground. Thirteen of the SSRD studies utilized frequency or interval counts of initiations and responses. As with the engagement method, definitions of initiations and responses often vary based on the coding system used in the study. For example, Barber, Saffo, Gilpin, Craft, and Goldstein (2016) defined an initiation as both nonverbal (e.g., bringing a toy to a peer) and verbal social bids toward peers, whereas Banda et al. (2010) included only verbal bids.

In five of the RCTs, live observation was used to measure children's initiations and responses. Live coding presents a number of challenges to researchers; the chaotic, loud, and dynamic environments of playgrounds and classrooms can make obtaining accurate estimates of children's true skills difficult.

4.5.5 Summary of Measures

A variety of assessments are used to measure the social communication skills and responses to intervention in children with ASD. Consideration of who is observing or reporting on the outcome (e.g., self-report, parents, teachers, blinded observers) and whether there is consistency across these reports is important when interpreting the results of an intervention. Direct observation and parent report measures are most commonly used, especially in studies of young children. Self-report measures are used less often but provide important information and perspective that may not be gleaned from other measurement techniques.

4.6 Study Findings

4.6.1 Single Subject Research Designs

The majority of the interventions (n = 13) utilized direct instruction with the child with ASD; that is, an adult models or teaches the child a skill and then the child must apply it to social situations with peers. These lessons included topics such as how to join a game, how to position ones' body when talking to a peer, and self-regulation. Eight of the studies utilized a peer-mediated approach where children's classmates, often neurotypical peers, were taught strategies to help facilitate social interactions with the children with ASD. These strategies included how to invite a peer with autism to join a game, how to resolve conflicts, and how to be persistent in the face of rejection. The primary difference between direct instruction and peer modeling is that the PMIs rely on an intermediary (peer models) to facilitate the target social skill rather than working directly with the children with ASD. These teaching strategies can be used in conjunction with each other; three of the studies utilized a combination of both direct instruction and PMIs and saw positive effects on children's outcomes (Banda et al., 2010; Laushey et al., 2009; Mason et al., 2014). A summary of the interventions and results can be found in Table 2.

The most common targets of intervention trials were social initiations to peers and appropriately responding to peers (n = 12). Many of the studies (n = 9) also targeted reciprocal social engagement (e.g., percentage of time engaged with peer) and some individualized the selection of the target social skill based on the needs of the child (e.g., Harper et al., 2008). For example, one child's target was gaining peers' attention, while another child's target was turn-taking with peers. In only a few instances (n = 5) were both frequency of social initiations (quantity) and engagement (quality) with peers measured (Koegel, Kuriakose, et al., 2012; Koegel, Vernon, et al., 2012; Koegel et al., 2014; Mundschenk & Sasso, 1995; Radley, Ford, Battaglia, & McHugh, 2014). Consideration of both the quantity and quality of social interactions is important. Increasing the frequency of engagement between peers may not be sufficient to build social connections and friendships. The quality of that engagement, such as having back-and-forth conversations, may be a critical component to improved social success within schools. To that end, two of the studies saw increases in engagement with peers without improvements in initiations (Koegel, Kuriakose, et al., 2012; Radley et al., 2014) showing that these targets are not intertwined and one can increase without the other. Interventions can increase children's engagement but additional support may be necessary for more challenging skills such as initiations.

Altogether, the SSRD studies demonstrated some increases in children's initiations and responses as well as engagement with peers. Looking first at initiations, 5 of the studies targeting initiations were found to have PND values falling in the effective range (Banda et al., 2010; Gena, 2006; Koegel, Vernon, et al., 2012; Koegel et al., 2014; Laushey et al., 2009) with the other 12 showing no evidence of treatment effects (e.g., Harper et al., 2008; Barber et al., 2016). PMIs (Brady, Shores, McEvoy, Ellis, & Fox, 1987; Harper et al., 2008; Owen-DeSchryver, Carr, Cale, & Blakeley-Smith, 2008) were not effective in targeting initiations with PND scores of 52%, 16%, and 59%, respectively. However, positive treatment effects of PMI were seen when this intervention was paired with direct instruction (Banda et al., 2010; Laushey et al., 2009). This finding may indicate that additional supported instructional time is needed for discrete skills such as initiations using peer-mediated models to be mastered and used in the dynamic context of real-world social interactions. However, due to the lack of replications of specific treatment techniques, it is difficult to determine whether the mixed and limited effects demonstrated across PMIs were seen as a result of variation in the intervention, based on broad treatment philosophies (e.g., direct instruction or peer-mediated), or can be explained by specific variations in study procedures (e.g., dose, fidelity, materials).

PND scores for four studies fell in the effective range in regards to improving children's responses to social bids (Banda et al., 2010; Barber et al., 2016; Gena, 2006; Laushey et al., 2009), while an equal number fell in the debatably effective or noneffective range (Mundschenk & Sasso, 1995; Owen-DeSchryver et al., 2008; Radley et al., 2014; Kamps et al., 2014). Responding was also sometimes captured amid other behaviors through the use of aggregate scores of social behaviors. These scores captured a number of different social behaviors, such as "communicative acts," which consist of both initiations and responses or "prosocial" behaviors such as sharing, initiating, and directing vocalizations toward peers. All of the studies using those measures met PND criteria for moderate effectiveness or higher (Laushey & Heflin, 2000; Mason et al., 2014; Shafer, Egel, & Neef, 1984) with the exception of one study which fell in the debatably effective range (Thiemann & Goldstein, 2004).

Lastly, looking at children's engagement or reciprocal interactions with peers, all (Feldman & Matos, 2013; Hartzell et al., 2015; Koegel et al., 2005, Koegel, Kuriakose, et al., 2012; Koegel, Vernon, et al., 2012; Koegel et al., 2014; Radley et al., 2014) except for one study (Mundschenk & Sasso, 1995) demonstrated results in the very effective range based on PND scores.

Of the 10 studies that measured maintenance of effects, through measuring their outcome in a follow-up period, six were successful (Brady et al., 1987; Feldman & Matos, 2013; Koegel, Kuriakose, et al., 2012; Koegel et al., 2014; Laushey et al., 2009; Wilson, 2013), and the remaining four had mixed results or unclear trends (Barber et al., 2016; Hartzell et al., 2015; Leaf et al., 2009; Thiemann & Goldstein, 2004). Looking next at whether the results generalized to a different setting, social partner, or interventionist, of the nine that measured generalization, seven were successful (Feldman & Matos, 2013; Harper et al., 2008; Hartzell et al., 2015; Kamps et al., 2014; Koegel, Kuriakose, et al., 2012; Laushey et al., 2009; Shafer et al., 1984) and two were not in generalizing the results (Gena, 2006; Owen-DeSchryver et al., 2008).

4.6.2 Randomized Controlled Trials

A full summary of the results of the RCTs included in the review can be found in Table 4. The most common metric to assess change in the primary outcome was direct observation of social behavior (n = 7). Half of the studies included a parent report measure of friendship quality, social acceptance, or social skills, while three included a measure of the teacher's perception of social skills, and six utilized self-report scores. Only half of the studies included a combination of an observational measure plus a report from the parent, teacher, or the child himself/herself. The use of multiple informants is important as discrepancies were seen between parent report scores and self-report (Koning et al., 2013) and between parent and teacher reports (Frankel et al., 2010; Young et al., 2016). These differences may reflect true differences in ability across contexts or may instead reflect differences in rater experiences and perspectives. Information on the included measures can be found in Table 4.

A number of promising effects were observed as a result of the intervention protocols evaluated in RCTs. A commonly addressed outcome was to examine engagement with peers (Kasari et al., 2016, 2012; Koning et al., 2013; Kretzmann et al., 2015; Wood et al., 2014). Several interventions measured gains in peer engagement including CBT (Koning et al., 2013; Wood et al., 2014), PMI (Kasari et al., 2012), didactic social skills groups (Kasari et al., 2016), and training paraprofessional aides to provide environmental support for children on the playground (Kretzmann et al., 2015).

The CBT approach showed mixed results, with one study (Wood et al., 2014) demonstrating large effects on peer engagement ($d = 1.36$) and the other (Koning et al., 2013) showing more modest effects (0.29). It is promising that playground staff were able to deliver an intervention successfully, leading to increases in children's engagement with a large effect size (Kretzmann et al., 2015) ($d = 1.27$).

Less consistent findings were seen in social network salience, but one PMI did find large treatment effects (Cohen's $d = 0.79$: Kasari et al., 2012). Studies that targeted broader social behaviors with norm-referenced measures (e.g., Kamps et al., 2015; Koning et al., 2013; Young et al., 2016), in general, saw smaller and less consistent effects. These norm-referenced measures represent more distal intervention targets (not directly targeted by the intervention) and therefore these small effects may be anticipated.

5. DISCUSSION

Establishing a clear understanding of the evidence supporting interventions targeting social skills and friendships in young children with ASD is essential. Across the studies including both SSRDs and RCTs, findings indicate that many interventions were successful in increasing children's social engagement with their peers. These positive results are promising; however, there are limitations to the current evidence that must be addressed. The following themes emerged from the review and include (1) the need to consider intervention approach when choosing treatment targets, (2) the choice of outcome measures and the validity of those measures, (3) the importance of external validity in social skills interventions, and (4) the directions for future research.

5.1 Intervention Approach

In both the RCT and SSRD studies, most interventions utilized direct instruction by a clinician, teacher, or paraprofessional within the school. Positive results were seen in peer-mediated models, and in a comparison of direct instruction to peer-mediated models, those receiving a PMI generally outperformed those who received only direct instruction across important outcomes such as friendship nominations, playground engagement, and social network salience (Kasari, et al., 2012). However, inconsistent results were seen in PMIs using SSRDs, especially for targeting discrete skills such as social initiations to peers. Generally, there were more positive results, based on an evaluation of the reported effect sizes, for discrete skills when peer-mediated and direct instructions were used together. It is unclear whether the observed differences are because of the specific intervention protocols used across trials, variation in the study samples, or other factors such as dose or context of the interventions. An important area of future research should be the replication of these results and further evaluation of the mechanisms of change within both the PMIs and direct instruction interventions that may lead to improved outcomes and how they may work synergistically. Further work to understand which treatment components are effective for which targets will increase our ability to apply effective interventions to more children. It is possible that the combination of peer-mediated and direct instruction are effective at teaching different skills, and reliance on only one method will not be effective for all children; but, to make these connections, future studies must use larger samples and rigorous methodologies.

Looking next at the treatment targets across treatment types, less consistent results were seen for discrete social skills such as initiating and responding to peers. One interpretation of this pattern is that it may be easier to increase the frequency and duration of social interactions through basic intervention strategies but improving the quality of these same interactions, such as increasing conversational turn-taking or the initiation of interactions, may require more intensive or individualized treatments. It may also be the case that more fleeting forms of engagement are easier to improve but sustained, quality interactions are more difficult. A careful consideration of the measures used is necessary to accurately evaluate the social engagement of children.

Specifically addressing the interventions that were tested using RCTs, there is evidence that many of the protocols that are "targeted" (e.g., intervene on specific skills) appear effective in improving outcomes. For example, Kretzmann et al. (2015) taught strategies to help playground aides facilitate play and saw increases in playground engagement. Kasari et al. (2012) taught peers strategies to engage children with ASD and saw increases in friendship nominations and peer engagement. Teacher-reported social skills were found to improve as a result of a comprehensive teacher-implemented intervention but there was no direct observation of social skills included (Young et al., 2016). These findings could be strengthened through direct observation of social connections with peers or friendships.

5.2 External Validity of Interventions

One common criticism of the interventions and treatment programs provided for children with ASD is that they take place within highly controlled settings (e.g., Barber et al., 2016) with one-on-one support from therapists. This raises the question of whether the skills taught within the intervention will generalize to complex and dynamic real-world social interactions with peers. It was therefore promising to see that almost all of the studies that were included in this review took place in schools (although the agent of implementation varied widely from trained clinicians to school staff such as aides and teachers), improving our confidence that the skills that are targeted may be directly related to better social outcomes for the children in their everyday social settings.

It is clear from the descriptive studies that children with ASD face many struggles as they navigate the complex social world within schools and that there are a number of barriers that make the implementation of interventions targeting peer engagement and friendship difficult within school contexts (where children spend much of their time) including staffing issues, competing demands of school staff, and the availability of resources to carry out research-based interventions (Locke et al., 2015). However, it was promising that some RCTs were implemented by school staff and saw positive effects on social communication outcomes and peer engagement (e.g., Kamps et al., 2015; Kretzmann et al., 2015; Young et al., 2016).

This improves confidence that interventions can be successfully transmitted to community settings when support is provided by research staff, increasing the impact of the interventions as they can reach more children.

Next, it is also important to note that while a majority of interventions took place in school, the degree to which the context of the intervention can be considered "natural" or "generalized" varies across studies. Some instruction took place in natural social contexts such as the playground using in vivo teaching (e.g., Mason et al., 2014), while other children received instruction in less generalized contexts such as pullout rooms or during class time (e.g., Owen-DeSchryver et al., 2008). Thus, even when some interventions took place in schools, they did not take advantage of opportunities for natural social interactions and teaching generalization. Of the 24 included SSRD studies, nine examined generalization. Of those studies, certain discrete skills, such as initiating to peers, appear to be more difficult for children to generalize (Harper et al., 2008; Kamps et al., 2014; Koegel, Kuriakose, et al., 2012) but overall, generalization probes were successful in the SSRDs in seven of the nine studies that measured it. That is, they were able to demonstrate the targeted skill in a different context than it was taught. This is promising as it points to children truly learning the targeted skill.

A majority (six of ten) of the SSRDs and five of six RCTs were successful (meaning, showing a statistically significant difference from entry to the follow-up period) in maintaining the gains made on the outcome during the intervention period. Many of the studies assessed maintenance through brief follow-up periods ranging from 2 weeks in some (e.g., Wilson, 2013) to 7 weeks in others (e.g., Feldman & Matos, 2013). Extending follow-up periods in future research could provide more clarity as to the lasting effects of the interventions, in particular, across school years. Only one trial (Kasari et al., 2012) measured skill retention across school years, so little is known about how these skills transfer to new peer groups or carry over across grades.

5.3 Future Directions

It is promising that several studies scored high on ratings of methodological quality that utilized RCTs (e.g., Koning et al., 2013) and SSRDs (e.g., Mason et al., 2014). Continued efforts should be made to address design elements such as blinding outcome assessors to condition/time/study hypothesis, demonstrating experimental control (at least three times within SSRDs), specifying a priori primary aims and their associated outcomes, as well as clearly describing the randomization procedures in text. Continued efforts to improve these components will allow greater confidence in the effectiveness of interventions to produce positive changes in friendships and social acceptance in children with ASD.

Poor social outcomes, including having fewer and lower quality friendships, less centrality to the social structure of their classes, poorer self-concept, and elevated feelings of loneliness are common among children with ASD. Despite these persistent findings, only three included studies directly examined friendships or social connections as outcomes. However, all three studies demonstrated some increases in friendships and social connections for children with ASD (Frankel et al., 2010; Kasari et al., 2016, 2012). The development of friendships is a meaningful treatment end point and positive results are noted when attempts were made to intervene on this target. As such, developing friendships and social connections should remain a central aim of future intervention research.

However, not all children with ASD have difficulty establishing friendships (Locke, Williams, Shih & Kasari, 2017). A small portion (around 10%) is popular in their classroom social structure. Understanding the strategies these children use may lead to the development of additional effective intervention practices. Among young children, children with friends tend to use more complex forms of nonverbal communication and are jointly engaged with peers at higher rates (Chang, Shih, & Kasari, 2016). Early joint attention is also linked to higher-quality friendships later in childhood (Freeman, Gulsrud, & Kasari, 2015). Therefore, joint attention skills and joint engagement may be important targets of interventions aimed at developing friendships and social connections in young children with ASD.

Even though observations of children's engagement are conducted based on both verbal and nonverbal behavior (e.g., eye contact, proximity, turns on a shared activity, joint attention gestures, etc.,), children who have limited language and cognitive skills are largely missing from this literature. A critical area of future research is to begin to understand friendships and social acceptance in children who have minimal spoken language and children with intellectual disability. Only two studies in the current review reported including children with a developmental level below 70 (Brady et al., 1987; Roeyers, 1996). To date, these groups of children have been largely left out of studies evaluating friendship and social connections. This may, in part, be due to the difficulty in assessing such a complex construct in a population of children who may not easily be able to report on their perceptions of friendship. However, the importance of companionship and friendship is clear and so efforts should be made to further understand this complex but clinically important domain in children with limited language and cognitive skills. The use of observational measures offers a method to evaluate various aspects of social interactions such as engagement and social initiations that may serve as appropriate proxies for companionship in certain cases if measured over time. The use of augmentative and alternative communication systems to increase social connectivity of children with ASD to their peers has shown some preliminary evidence of effectiveness (Kravits, Kamps, Kemmerer, & Potucek, 2002; Trembath, Balandin, Togher, & Stancliffe, 2009), although more research is needed to draw definitive conclusions.

5.4 Limitations

An important limitation of this review to note is the utilization of PND as the effect size metric for SSRD. There is no single agreed on metric to evaluate the effect sizes of SSRDs and results may change if another method was used (e.g., percentage of data exceeding the median or all PND). A consideration of the data from each individual study is needed to make an appropriate choice of estimate (Lenz, 2013); this is not possible in the context of a review.

6. CONCLUSIONS

While some limitations remain in the current literature, there were a number of positive themes that emerged from this review. The first, being the focus on the external validity and generalizability of intervention outcomes. Next, being the consistent positive effects seen on some child outcomes such as engagement. Last, being the increased methodological rigor seen in some trials that give more confidence in interpreting the data. Further research is needed to both refine and replicate the results shown in these trials. Directions for future research include targeting proximal outcomes known to have distal effects on important child outcomes such as friendship development and social acceptance, the inclusion of more diverse clinical populations, including those who have complex communication needs and an increased focus on implementing interventions that are sustainable and effective in real-world context. With these goals in mind, the next generation of intervention research will continue to promote the successful social inclusion of children with ASD within schools.

REFERENCES

Adamson, L. B., Bakeman, R., Deckner, D. F., & Romski, M. (2009). Joint engagement and the emergence of language in children with autism and Down syndrome. *Journal of Autism and Developmental Disorders, 39*(1), 84.

American Psychiatric Association. (2013). *Diagnostic and statistical manual of mental disorders (DSM-5®)*. American Psychiatric Pub.

Anderson, A., Locke, J., Kretzmann, M., Kasari, C., & Network, A. B. (2015). Social network analysis of children with autism spectrum disorder: Predictors of fragmentation and connectivity in elementary school classrooms. *Autism*. http://dx.doi.org/10.1177/1362361315603568.

Banda, D. R., Hart, S. L., & Liu-Gitz, L. (2010). Impact of training peers and children with autism on social skills during center time activities in inclusive classrooms. *Research in Autism Spectrum Disorders, 4*(4), 619–625.

Barber, A. B., Saffo, R. W., Gilpin, A. T., Craft, L. D., & Goldstein, H. (2016). Peers as clinicians: Examining the impact of Stay Play Talk on social communication in young preschoolers with autism. *Journal of Communication Disorders, 59*, 1–15.

Barry, T. D., Klinger, L. G., Lee, J. M., Palardy, N., Gilmore, T., & Bodin, S. D. (2003). Examining the effectiveness of an outpatient clinic–based social skills group for high-functioning children with autism. *Journal of Autism and Developmental Disorders, 33*(6), 685–701.

Bauminger, N., & Kasari, C. (2000). Loneliness and friendship in high-functioning children with autism. *Child development, 71*(2), 447–456.

Bauminger, N., Shulman, C., & Agam, G. (2003). Peer interaction and loneliness in high-functioning children with autism. *Journal of Autism and Developmental Disorders, 33*(5), 489–507.

Brady, M. P., Shores, R. E., McEvoy, M. A., Ellis, D., & Fox, J. J. (1987). Increasing social interactions of severely handicapped autistic children. *Journal of Autism and Developmental Disorders, 17*(3), 375–390.

Bukowski, W. M., Hoza, B., & Boivin, M. (1994). Measuring friendship quality during pre-and early adolescence: The development and psychometric properties of the friendship qualities scale. *Journal of Social and Personal Relationships, 11*(3), 471–484.

Cairns, R. B., Cairns, B. D., Neckerman, H. J., Gest, S. D., & Gariepy, J. L. (1988). Social networks and aggressive behavior: Peer support or peer rejection? *Developmental Psychology, 24*(6), 815.

Chamberlain, B., Kasari, C., & Rotheram-Fuller, E. (2007). Involvement or isolation? The social networks of children with autism in regular classrooms. *Journal of Autism and Developmental Disorders, 37*(2), 230–242.

Chang, Y. C., Shih, W., & Kasari, C. (2016). Friendships in preschool children with autism spectrum disorder: What holds them back, child characteristics or teacher behavior? *Autism, 20*(1), 65–74.

Constantino, J. N., Davis, S. A., Todd, R. D., Schindler, M. K., Gross, M. M., Brophy, S. L., … Reich, W. (2003). Validation of a brief quantitative measure of autistic traits: Comparison of the social responsiveness scale with the autism diagnostic interview-revised. *Journal of Autism and Developmental Disorders, 33*(4), 427–433.

Dawson, G., Toth, K., Abbott, R., Osterling, J., Munson, J., Estes, A., & Liaw, J. (2004). Early social attention impairments in autism: Social orienting, joint attention, and attention to distress. *Developmental Psychology, 40*(2), 271.

Dean, M., Harwood, R., & Kasari, C. (2016). The art of camouflage: Gender differences in the social behaviors of girls and boys with autism spectrum disorder. *Autism*. http://dx.doi.org/10.1177/1362361316671845.

Dean, M., Kasari, C., Shih, W., Frankel, F., Whitney, R., , ... Landa, R., & Harwood, R. (2014). The peer relationships of girls with ASD at school: Comparison to boys andgirls with and without ASD. *Journal of Child Psychology and Psychiatry, 55*(11), 1218–1225.
Feldman, E. K., & Matos, R. (2013). Training paraprofessionals to facilitate social interactions between children with autism and their typically developing peers. *Journal of Positive Behavior Interventions, 15*(3), 169–179.
Frankel, F., Myatt, R., Sugar, C., Whitham, C., Gorospe, C. M., & Laugeson, E. (2010). A randomized controlled study of parent-assisted children's friendship training with children having autism spectrum disorders. *Journal of Autism and Developmental Disorders, 40*(7), 827–842.
Freeman, S. F., Gulsrud, A., & Kasari, C. (2015). Brief report: Linking early joint attention and play abilities to later reports of friendships for children with ASD. *Journal of Autism and Developmental Disorders, 45*(7), 2259–2266.
Gena, A. (2006). The effects of prompting and social reinforcement on establishing social interactions with peers during the inclusion of four children with autism in preschool. *International Journal of Psychology, 41*(6), 541–554.
Gonzalez-Lopez, A., & Kamps, D. M. (1997). Social skills training to increase social interactions between children with autism and their typical peers. *Focus on Autism and Other Developmental Disabilities, 12*(1), 2–14.
Green, J., Charman, T., McConachie, H., Aldred, C., Slonims, V., Howlin, P., ... Barrett, B. (2010). Parent-mediated communication-focused treatment in children with autism (PACT): A randomised controlled trial. *Lancet, 375*(9732), 2152–2160.
Hardan, A. Y., Gengoux, G. W., Berquist, K. L., Libove, R. A., Ardel, C. M., Phillips, J., ... Minjarez, M. B. (2015). A randomized controlled trial of Pivotal Response Treatment Group for parents of children with autism. *Journal of Child Psychology and Psychiatry, 56*(8), 884–892.
Harper, C. B., Symon, J. B., & Frea, W. D. (2008). Recess is time-in: Using peers to improve social skills of children with autism. *Journal of Autism and Developmental Disorders, 38*(5), 815–826.
Hartzell, R., Liaupsin, C., Gann, C., & Clem, S. (2015). Increasing social engagement in an inclusive environment. *Education and Training in Autism and Developmental Disabilities, 50*(3), 264.
Hauck, M., Fein, D., Waterhouse, L., & Feinstein, C. (1995). Social initiations by autistic children to adults and other children. *Journal of Autism and Developmental Disorders, 25*(6), 579–595.
Higgins, J. P. T., & Green, S. (Eds.). (2011). Cochrane handbook for systematic reviews of interventions (Version 5.1.0, updated March 2011). The Cochrane Collaboration. Available from www.handbook.cochrane.org.
Hodges, E. V., Boivin, M., Vitaro, F., & Bukowski, W. M. (1999). The power of friendship: Protection against an escalating cycle of peer victimization. *Developmental Psychology, 35*(1), 94.
Kamps, D., Mason, R., Thiemann-Bourque, K., Feldmiller, S., Turcotte, A., & Miller, T. (2014). The use of peer networks to increase communicative acts of students with autism spectrum disorders. *Focus on Autism and Other Developmental Disabilities, 29*(4), 230–245.
Kamps, D., Thiemann-Bourque, K., Heitzman-Powell, L., Schwartz, I., Rosenberg, N., Mason, R., & Cox, S. (2015). A comprehensive peer network intervention to improve social communication of children with autism spectrum disorders: A randomized trial in kindergarten and first grade. *Journal of Autism and Developmental Disorders, 45*(6), 1809–1824.
Kanner, L. (1943). *Autistic disturbances of affective contact.*
Kasari, C., Dean, M., Kretzmann, M., Shih, W., Orlich, F., Whitney, R., ... King, B. (2016). Children with autism spectrum disorder and social skills groups at school: A randomized trial comparing intervention approach and peer composition. *Journal of Child Psychology and Psychiatry, 57*(2), 171–179.

Kasari, C., Freeman, S., & Paparella, T. (2006). Joint attention and symbolic play in young children with autism: A randomized controlled intervention study. *Journal of Child Psychology and Psychiatry, 47*(6), 611–620.

Kasari, C., Gulsrud, A., Paparella, T., Hellemann, G., & Berry, K. (2015). Randomized comparative efficacy study of parent-mediated interventions for toddlers with autism. *Journal of Consulting and Clinical Psychology, 83*(3), 554.

Kasari, C., Locke, J., Gulsrud, A., & Rotheram-Fuller, E. (2011). Social networks and friendships at school: Comparing children with and without ASD. *Journal of Autism and Developmental Disorders, 41*(5), 533–544.

Kasari, C., Rotheram-Fuller, E., Locke, J., & Gulsrud, A. (2012). Making the connection: Randomized controlled trial of social skills at school for children with autism spectrum disorders. *Journal of Child Psychology and Psychiatry, 53*(4), 431–439.

Kasari, C., & Rotheram-Fuller, L. J. (2005). *The development of the playground observation of peer engagement (POPE) Measure*. Los Angeles, CA: University of California Los Angeles. Unpublished manuscript.

Koegel, L. K., Kuriakose, S., Singh, A. K., & Koegel, R. L. (2012). Improving generalization of peer socialization gains in inclusive school settings using initiations training. *Behavior Modification, 36*(3), 361–377.

Koegel, L. K., Vernon, T. W., Koegel, R. L., Koegel, B. L., & Paullin, A. W. (2012). Improving social engagement and initiations between children with autism spectrum disorder and their peers in inclusive settings. *Journal of Positive Behavior Interventions, 14*(4), 220–227.

Koegel, R. L., Kim, S., & Koegel, L. K. (2014). Training paraprofessionals to improve socialization in students with ASD. *Journal of Autism and Developmental Disorders, 44*(9), 2197–2208.

Koegel, R. L., Werner, G. A., Vismara, L. A., & Koegel, L. K. (2005). The effectiveness of contextually supported play date interactions between children with autism and typically developing peers. *Research and Practice for Persons with Severe Disabilities, 30*(2), 93–102.

Koning, C., Magill-Evans, J., Volden, J., & Dick, B. (2013). Efficacy of cognitive behavior therapy-based social skills intervention for school-aged boys with autism spectrum disorders. *Research in Autism Spectrum Disorders,* 7(10), 1282–1290.

Kravits, T. R., Kamps, D. M., Kemmerer, K., & Potucek, J. (2002). Brief report: Increasing communication skills for an elementary-aged student with autism using the picture exchange communication system. *Journal of Autism and Developmental Disorders, 32*(3), 225–230.

Kretzmann, M., Shih, W., & Kasari, C. (2015). Improving peer engagement of children with autism on the school playground: A randomized controlled trial. *Behavior Therapy, 46*(1), 20–28.

Ladd, G. W., Kochenderfer, B. J., & Coleman, C. C. (1996). Friendship quality as a predictor of young children's early school adjustment. *Child Development, 67*(3), 1103–1118.

Laushey, K. M., & Heflin, L. J. (2000). Enhancing social skills of kindergarten children with autism through the training of multiple peers as tutors. *Journal of Autism and Developmental Disorders, 30*(3), 183–193.

Laushey, K. M., Heflin, L. J., Shippen, M., Alberto, P. A., & Fredrick, L. (2009). Concept mastery routines to teach social skills to elementary children with high functioning autism. *Journal of Autism and Developmental Disorders, 39*(10), 1435–1448.

Le Couteur, A., Lord, C., & Rutter, M. (2003). *The autism diagnostic interview-revised (ADI-R)*. Los Angeles, CA: Western Psychological Services.

Leaf, J. B., Taubman, M., Bloomfield, S., Palos-Rafuse, L., Leaf, R., McEachin, J., & Oppenheim, M. L. (2009). Increasing social skills and pro-social behavior for three children diagnosed with autism through the use of a teaching package. *Research in Autism Spectrum Disorders, 3*(1), 275–289.

Lenz, A. S. (2013). Calculating effect size in single-case research: A comparison of nonoverlap methods. *Measurement and Evaluation in Counseling and Development, 46*(1), 64–73.
Locke, J., Kasari, C., Rotheram-Fuller, E., Kretzmann, M., & Jacobs, J. (2013). Social network changes over the school year among elementary school-aged children with and without an autism spectrum disorder. *School Mental Health, 5*(1), 38–47.
Locke, J., Olsen, A., Wideman, R., Downey, M. M., Kretzmann, M., Kasari, C., & Mandell, D. S. (2015). A tangled web: The challenges of implementing an evidence-based social engagement intervention for children with autism in urban public school settings. *Behavior Therapy, 46*(1), 54–67.
Locke, J., Williams, J., Shih, W., & Kasari, C. (2017). Characteristics of socially successful elementary school-aged children with autism. *Journal of Child Psychology and Psychiatry, 58*(1), 94–102.
Logan, L. R., Hickman, R. R., Harris, S. R., & Heriza, C. B. (2008). Single-subject research design: Recommendations for levels of evidence and quality rating. *Developmental Medicine & Child Neurology, 50*(2), 99–103.
Lord, C., Rutter, M., DiLavore, P. C., Risi, S., Gotham, K., & Bishop, S. (2012). *Autism diagnostic observation schedule: ADOS-2*. Los Angeles, CA: Western Psychological Services.
Mandell, D. S., Stahmer, A. C., Shin, S., Xie, M., Reisinger, E., & Marcus, S. C. (2013). The role of treatment fidelity on outcomes during a randomized field trial of an autism intervention. *Autism, 17*(3), 281–295.
Margalit, M. (2012). *Loneliness among children with special needs: Theory, research, coping, and intervention*. Springer Science & Business Media.
Mason, R., Kamps, D., Turcotte, A., Cox, S., Feldmiller, S., & Miller, T. (2014). Peer mediation to increase communication and interaction at recess for students with autism spectrum disorders. *Research in Autism Spectrum Disorders, 8*(3), 334–344.
Mundschenk, N. A., & Sasso, G. M. (1995). Assessing sufficient social exemplars for students with autism. *Behavioral Disorders*, 62–78.
Odom, S. L., McConnell, S. R., Ostrosky, M., Peterson, C., Skellenger, A., Spicuzza, R., … McEvoy, M. A. (1997). *Play time/social Time: Organizing your classroom to build interaction skills*.
Oono, I. P., Honey, E. J., & McConachie, H. (2013). Parent-mediated early intervention for young children with autism spectrum disorders (ASD). *Evidence-Based Child Health: A Cochrane Review Journal, 8*(6), 2380–2479.
Owen-DeSchryver, J. S., Carr, E. G., Cale, S. I., & Blakeley-Smith, A. (2008). Promoting social interactions between students with autism spectrum disorders and their peers in inclusive school settings. *Focus on Autism and Other Developmental Disabilities, 23*(1), 15–28.
Ozonoff, S., & Miller, J. N. (1995). Teaching theory of mind: A new approach to social skills training for individuals with autism. *Journal of Autism and Developmental Disorders, 25*(4), 415–433.
Palomo, R., Belinchón, M., & Ozonoff, S. (2006). Autism and family home movies: A comprehensive review. *Journal of Developmental & Behavioral Pediatrics, 27*(2), S59–S68.
Parker, J. G., Saxon, J. L., Asher, S. R., & Kovacs, D. M. (1999). Dimensions of children's friendship adjustment: Implications for understanding loneliness. *Loneliness in Childhood and Adolescence*, 201–221.
Radley, K. C., Ford, W. B., Battaglia, A. A., & McHugh, M. B. (2014). The effects of a social skills training package on social engagement of children with autism spectrum disorders in a generalized recess setting. *Focus on Autism and Other Developmental Disabilities, 29*.
Roeyers, H. (1996). The influence of nonhandicapped peers on the social interactions of children with a pervasive developmental disorder. *Journal of Autism and Developmental Disorders, 26*(3), 303–320.

Rosenberg, N., Congdon, M., Schwartz, I., & Kamps, D. (2015). Use of say-do correspondence training to increase generalization of social interaction skills at recess for children with autism spectrum disorder. *Education and Training in Autism and Developmental Disabilities, 50*(2), 213.

Rotheram-Fuller, E., Kasari, C., Chamberlain, B., & Locke, J. (2010). Social involvement of children with autism spectrum disorders in elementary school classrooms. *Journal of Child Psychology and Psychiatry, 51*(11), 1227–1234.

Rubin, K. H., LeMare, L. J., & Lollis, S. (1990). Social withdrawal in childhood: Developmental pathways to peer rejection. *Peer Rejection in Childhood*, 217–249.

Scruggs, T. E., & Mastropieri, M. A. (1998). Summarizing single-subject research: Issues and applications. *Behavior Modification, 22*(3), 221–242.

Shafer, M. S., Egel, A. L., & Neef, N. A. (1984). Training mildly handicapped peers to facilitate changes in the social interaction skills of autistic children. *Journal of Applied Behavior Analysis, 17*(4), 461–476.

Sigman, M., Ruskin, E., Arbelle, S., Corona, R., Dissanayake, C., Espinosa, M., … Robinson, B. F. (1999). Continuity and change in the social competence of children with autism, Down syndrome, and developmental delays. *Monographs of the Society for Research in Child Development*, 1–139.

Soorya, L. V., Siper, P. M., Beck, T., Soffes, S., Halpern, D., Gorenstein, M., … Wang, A. T. (2015). Randomized comparative trial of a social cognitive skills group for children with autism spectrum disorder. *Journal of the American Academy of Child and Adolescent Psychiatry, 54*(3), 208–216.

Spitzberg, B. H., & Hurt, H. T. (1987). The relationship of interpersonal competence and skills to reported loneliness across time. *Journal of Social Behavior and Personality, 2*(2), 157.

Stahmer, A. C., Rieth, S., Lee, E., Reisinger, E. M., Mandell, D. S., & Connell, J. E. (2015). Training teachers to use evidence-based practices for autism: Examining procedural implementation fidelity. *Psychology in the Schools, 52*(2), 181–195.

Thiemann, K. S., & Goldstein, H. (2004). Effects of peer training and written text cueing on social communication of school-age children with pervasive developmental disorder. *Journal of Speech, Language, and Hearing Research, 47*(1), 126–144.

Travis, L. L., & Sigman, M. (1998). Social deficits and interpersonal relationships in autism. *Developmental Disabilities Research Reviews, 4*(2), 65–72.

Trembath, D., Balandin, S., Togher, L., & Stancliffe, R. J. (2009). Peer-mediated teaching and augmentative and alternative communication for preschool-aged children with autism. *Journal of Intellectual & Developmental Disability, 34*(2), 173–186.

Volkmar, F., Carter, A., Grossman, J., & Klin, A. (1997). Social development in autism. *Handbook of Autism and Pervasive Developmental Disorders, 2*, 173–194.

Wilson, K. P. (2013). Teaching social-communication skills to preschoolers with autism: Efficacy of video versus in vivo modeling in the classroom. *Journal of Autism and Developmental Disorders, 43*(8), 1819–1831.

Wood, J. J., Fujii, C., Renno, P., & Van Dyke, M. (2014). Impact of cognitive behavioral therapy on observed autism symptom severity during school recess: A preliminary randomized, controlled trial. *Journal of Autism and Developmental Disorders, 44*(9), 2264–2276.

Young, H. E., Falco, R. A., & Hanita, M. (2016). Randomized, controlled trial of a comprehensive program for young students with autism spectrum disorder. *Journal of Autism and Developmental Disorders, 46*(2), 544–560.

CHAPTER THREE

Negative Peer Experiences in Adolescents With Autism Spectrum Disorders

Ryan Adams*[,1], **Somer Bishop**[§], **Julie Lounds Taylor**[¶]
*Cincinnati Children's Hospital Medical Center, Cincinnati, OH, United States
[§]University of California—San Francisco, San Francisco, CA, United States
[¶]Vanderbilt University Medical Center, Nashville, TN, United States
[1]Corresponding author: E-mail: Ryan.Adams@cchmc.org

Contents

Abstract

This chapter examines negative peer experiences (e.g., peer victimization, being ignored or excluded, and direct and indirect rejection) in adolescents with autism spectrum disorders (ASD). Discussion is concentrated on adolescents with higher cognitive and language abilities, with a focus on providing insights and suggestions for the next phase of studies that will inform interventions targeting negative experiences in this group. The chapter describes negative peer experiences in terms of nomenclature,

International Review of Research in Developmental Disabilities, Volume 52
ISSN 2211-6095
http://dx.doi.org/10.1016/bs.irrdd.2017.07.003

general findings, and important issues for adolescents with ASD; identifies common methodological issues with previous studies on this topic; presents a study on the impact of peer victimization in adolescents with ASD using obese adolescents as a comparison group; and finally, provides suggestions for advancing research in this topic area.

Given that autism spectrum disorders (ASD) are characterized by deficits in social communication, social cognition, and social motivation, it is not surprising that difficulties in the peer group are exceedingly common for adolescents with ASD. Parent-reported rates of peer victimization in individuals with ASD have been shown to range from 40% to 90% (Cappadocia, Weiss, & Pepler, 2012; Little, 2002; Maiano, Normand, Salvas, Moullec, & Aime, 2016; Sterzing, Shattuck, Narendorf, Wagner, & Cooper, 2012), surpassing rates seen in typically developing (TD) adolescents (Bear, Mantz, Glutting, Yang, & Boyer, 2015; Humphrey & Symes, 2011; Rose, Simpson, & Moss, 2015; Rowley et al., 2012; Twyman et al., 2010; Wainscot, Naylor, Sutcliffe, Tantam, & Williams, 2008; Zeedyk, Rodriguez, Tipton, Baker, & Blacher, 2014) and those with other disabilities (Humphrey & Symes, 2011; Rowley et al., 2012; Twyman et al., 2010; Zeedyk et al., 2014).

The reason that these youths are at risk is, at least in part, because of the symptoms and characteristics associated with ASD itself. Symptoms of ASD, and associated behaviors that are common among individuals with ASD (e.g., hyperactivity, aggression, poor emotion regulation) have been found to increase the likelihood of negative peer experiences (Card & Little, 2006). The presence of internalizing problems, which is another common problem for adolescents with ASD, also increases the likelihood of being a target of victimization. Moreover, internalizing symptoms also make these individuals more susceptible to the negative outcomes of difficult peer experiences (Card & Little, 2006; Reijntjes, Kamphuis, Prinzie, & Telch, 2010).

ASD-related symptoms and comorbidities increase vulnerability to the negative effects resulting from these experiences in additional ways. For example, social deficits characteristic of ASD (e.g., difficulty forming and maintaining friendships) make it less likely that adolescents with ASD can benefit from the positive effects of friendships and peer acceptance. Friendships and peer acceptance have been shown to protect TD adolescents from being targets of negative peer experiences (Hodges, Malone, & Perry, 1997; Hodges, Boivin, Vitaro, & Bukowski, 1999), as well as protect against the adverse outcomes resulting from negative peer experiences (Adams & Cantin, 2013; Adams, Santo, & Bukowski, 2011; Hodges et al., 1999; Prinstein, Boergers, & Vernberg, 2001). Finally, ASD symptoms could decrease the effectiveness of interventions, as difficulties with generalization and social insight might limit the abilities of youth with ASD to utilize strategies effective in reducing negative peer experiences among TD adolescents (Kärnä et al., 2013; A. Kärnä, M. Voeten, T. D. Little, E. Poskiparta, E. Alanen et al., 2011).

In light of the high rates of negative peer experiences reported in adolescents with ASD, as well as the almost certain negative impact of these experiences on development, there is clearly a need for interventions to address this problem. However, there are currently no empirically validated interventions for adolescents with ASD. The dearth of interventions for this group is most likely due to the lack of information that is needed to be able to develop effective interventions. As will be discussed in more detail below, we lack information about peer experiences required for creating successful interventions for these adolescents. In this respect, what follows is not a comprehensive review of the literature on peer experiences in ASD, but rather an overview of the issues that must be considered in future studies on this topic.

Toward providing information to inform such studies, we describe negative peer experiences for adolescents with ASD by providing definitions and distinctions between the various types of negative peer experiences and what is known about this group's general treatment in the peer world. Next, we outline various methodological issues that have hindered the interpretation of previous studies on this topic and provide recommendations for addressing these issues. Then, we provide evidence for the impact of peer victimization on adolescents with ASD by comparing adolescents with ASD to a new comparison group, adolescents who are obese, that hold clear evidence of the impact of peer victimization. Finally, we provide suggestions for topics that future studies should address when examining negative peer experiences to provide the findings needed to inform successful interventions. As discussed below, this chapter will focus on studies of adolescents with ASD with higher cognitive and language abilities.

1. A SPECIAL FOCUS ON HIGHER FUNCTIONING ADOLESCENTS WITH AUTISM SPECTRUM DISORDERS

The focus of the current chapter is on the developmental period of adolescence, and more specifically, on adolescents with ASD with higher cognitive and language abilities. This developmental period is particularly important since it is a time when expanded autonomy is coupled with changes in the social world, resulting in more time being spent in the peer world, as well as a broader range of social experiences and interaction partners. Changes in the social world that occur during adolescence increase the level of difficulty of social interactions, which requires increased sophistication in social skills and understanding that is lacking for many adolescents with ASD. This places adolescents with ASD at even higher risk for negative interactions.

The complexity of social experiences during this developmental period compared to earlier periods means that studies and interventions targeting peer experiences must recognize and account for developmental differences in the etiology, meaning, and outcomes of peer experiences that are specific to adolescence. For instance, physical aggression that occurs between two 5-year-olds is very different than physical aggression between two 16-year-olds. Recognizing developmental differences in social experiences is necessary so that interventions can be designed to actually address the specific experiences that are most salient or troublesome during adolescence.

The higher risk for negative peer experiences during this period of development also makes adolescence a critical window for providing interventions (Nansel et al., 2001). Timing interventions to occur early in adolescence could help to reduce the likelihood of negative experiences before risk factors increasing the likelihood of negative experiences become fully realized. For example, if we see increases in rates of these experiences just after entering high school, interventions could be started during high school, and these interventions could be tailored to address the specific types of experiences that are most salient at this time. Additionally, adolescence can be an ideal time to deliver interventions that aim to provide targeted social skill and social cognitive training because it precedes the transition to young adulthood, at which point individuals with ASD lose access to many of the supports and services available through the school system (Taylor & Mailick, 2014; Taylor et al., 2012). Thus, interventions can be implemented in middle and high school, while there are still resources available to help promote a more successful transition into the adult social world.

In addition to focusing on adolescence, this chapter is specifically concerned with adolescents with ASD with higher cognitive and language abilities. Individuals with ASD who have fluent language are more likely to spend time in regular education settings, as well as in other settings outside of the classroom that have less adult supervision. This increases the likelihood of encountering negative peer experiences, because it is more difficult for adults to monitor their social interactions (Nishina & Bellmore, 2010). Mainstreamed students with ASD are less liked by peers and more likely to be rejected, ignored, and purposely excluded by the peer group in comparison to their TD classmates (Bauminger & Kasari, 2000; Chamberlain, Kasari, & Rotheram-Fuller, 2007; Humphrey & Symes, 2010; Jones & Frederickson, 2010; Locke, Ishijima, Kasari, & London, 2010; Lyons, Cappadocia, & Weiss, 2011; Petrina, Carter, & Stephenson, 2014; Symes & Humphrey, 2010). Typical peers in general education classrooms report that they would be less likely to want to work or play with their ASD classmates compared with TD classmates. Students with ASD in these classrooms report receiving less support from their classmates, spend more time in solitary activities, and spend less time in cooperative interactions with classmates (Humphrey & Symes, 2010; Symes & Humphrey, 2010). They have fewer friendship nominations, fewer reciprocated friendships, spend less time with friends, and have lower friendship quality compared with TD classmates (Bauminger & Kasari, 2000; Lyons et al., 2011; Petrina et al., 2014).

When considered together, it should not be surprising that this group also reports higher rates of loneliness than their TD classmates (Chamberlain et al., 2007; Locke et al., 2010). Thus, in addition to being at greater risk for negative peer experiences, this group might also be more negatively affected by negative experiences than adolescents with lower cognitive and language abilities. "Higher functioning" youth are not only more likely to recognize negative experiences when they occur, but they are also more capable of recognizing differences between themselves and typical peers, both which place them at higher risk for internalizing problems (Ghaziuddin, Ghaziuddin, & Greden, 2002).

It is important to note that a focus on adolescents with higher cognitive and language abilities does not mean that those with intellectual disabilities and/or minimal verbal abilities do not also experience problems in the peer world. Rather, by first addressing the complexities and the wider range of experiences relevant for adolescents with higher cognitive and language abilities, it is our hope that the insights resulting from this work could be used to inform intervention development for individuals with ASD and non-ASD diagnoses of different ages and cognitive ability levels.

2. DESCRIBING NEGATIVE PEER EXPERIENCES FOR ADOLESCENTS WITH AUTISM SPECTRUM DISORDERS

This chapter examines a range of negative experiences, including different types of peer victimization (i.e., verbal, relational, physical), as well as being actively rejected (which is not mutually exclusive from peer victimization), passively excluded, and actively ignored. Studies in the TD population show that interventions targeting negative peer experiences are most successful when they provide specific strategies to target specific types of negative experiences (Kärnä et al., 2013, A. Kärnä, M. Voeten, T. D. Little, E. Poskiparta, E. Alanen et al., 2011). However, many current interventions for both TD and ASD adolescents are quite broad and address many forms of negative experiences in a way that does not distinguish between the various types of experiences. These interventions utilize vague strategies (e.g., "stand up to bullying") that are often unsuccessful (Polanin, Espelage, & Pigott, 2012; Yeager, Fong, Lee, & Espelage, 2015). To be effective, interventions must provide prevention strategies that are specific to each form of experience (Kärnä et al., 2013, A. Kärnä, M. Voeten, T. D. Little, E. Poskiparta, E. Alanen et al., 2011).

Along with distinguishing between types negative peer experiences, it is also important to distinguish between various forms of peer victimization. For instance, strategies for addressing physical peer victimization are not appropriate for addressing verbal victimization, and some strategies for addressing verbal victimization are not effective for addressing being ignored. Different various forms of peer victimization are also associated with different outcomes and predictors. In studies of TD adolescents, verbal victimization has the highest rates, followed by relational forms of peer victimization (e.g., gossip, saying mean things about them behind their backs, excluding from a group), and physical forms have the lowest rates. In contrast to the plethora of studies addressing different forms of peer victimization in TD adolescents, there are only a few studies of individuals with ASD that distinguish between types of peer victimization (e.g., Adams, Fredstrom, Duncan, Holleb, & Bishop, 2014; Bear et al., 2015; Kloosterman, Kelley, Craig, Parker, & Javier, 2013; Maiano et al., 2016; Nowell, Brewton, & Goin-Kochel, 2014; Wainscot et al., 2008; Zeedyk et al., 2014). In our own study of peer victimization of adolescents with ASD in general education classrooms (Adams et al., 2014), we found a similar pattern as seen in studies of TD adolescents, with both self-report and parent report indicating highest to lowest rates for verbal, relational, and physical victimization.

Most studies of negative peer experiences focus on peer victimization. However, other types of negative experiences, such as being left out, being looked over for peer activities, and being ignored, can be just as detrimental to health and well-being (Bowker, Adams, Fredstrom, & Gilman, 2014). Given what is known about limited social interactions and lack of friendships in individuals with ASD (Bauminger & Kasari, 2000; Lyons et al., 2011; Petrina et al., 2014), these types of experiences may be especially common for adolescents with ASD. In some cases, behaviors that adolescents with ASD exhibit can result in being targeted for peer victimization, but it may also be just as likely that these behaviors result in being left out or actively ignored. For example, many adolescents with ASD exhibit behaviors that peers may not understand or may see as negative or inappropriate. In turn, their peers may think that not including or ignoring such an individual is better than actively rejecting him/her through peer victimization. It is also common for adults to advise adolescents to "ignore" or to not engage someone who is difficult or confusing. TD adolescents might also passively exclude their peers with ASD because they do not know how to interact with individuals with ASD and are afraid of doing something wrong.

Being ignored and excluded has direct negative effects on well-being (Bowker et al., 2014; Gooren, van Lier, Stegge, Terwogt, & Koot, 2011; Williams, 2007); it also has indirect effects on other outcomes by depriving these individuals of positive peer experiences and relationships. Research in TD groups has shown that positive peer behaviors and friendships buffer the adverse effects of negative peer experiences, and provide protection against being victimized (Adams & Cantin, 2013; Adams et al., 2011; Hodges et al., 1997, 1999; Prinstein et al., 2001). Thus, individuals that are ignored or left out are indirectly put at risk for further peer victimization (and related negative outcomes) since they are less likely to benefit from protective factors.

3. METHODOLOGICAL ISSUES TO ADDRESS

In this section, we provide recommendations for addressing methodological issues that, in our opinion, are commonly found in studies of negative peer experiences in ASD and also raise some of the largest concerns for interpreting the findings from these studies. These comments are not intended to criticize studies conducted in the past, and in fact some of our own studies are guilty of not following best practices for measuring negative peer experiences. Research on peer problems in ASD—particularly during adolescence and beyond—is relatively new. Thus, like any other field of study in its early stages, researchers have had to deal with limited resources in conducting research in this area.

This lack of resources has led researchers to conduct retrospective data analyses on previously collected datasets, or to "slip" a few peer measures into studies not focused on peer issues. The limitations inherent in such studies have forced many to make less than ideal methodological choices when testing questions about peer experiences. For instance, because many studies take data from studies that did not incorporate measures specific to peer issues, researchers have had to rely on single-item measures of negative peer experiences. As we detail below, this approach raises many methodological concerns.

The following section outlines some common methodological issues that should be addressed as the field moves forward. In our opinion, methodological issues have limited the interpretation, and in turn, the impact of the current pool of findings from past studies on negative peer experiences of those with ASD. These issues may be the source of incongruent findings on this topic. For instance, we find a wide range of rates for peer victimization/bullying across studies, with rates of "bullying" ranging from 40% to 94% (Cappadocia et al., 2012; Little, 2002; Sterzing et al., 2012). Various methodological issues described below may help to explain such a wide range. These concerns also open up findings from previous studies to possible alternative interpretations and could affect the power to detect the effects under study, making it difficult to garner insights needed to build effective interventions.

3.1 Self-Reports

Studies of TD adolescents have found that, in comparison to other reports, self-reports of negative peer experiences are better predictors of some outcomes, such as internalizing problems (Adams & Cantin, 2013; Juvonen, Nishina, & Graham, 2001). This suggests that self-reports are important for understanding the effects of negative peer experience. Self-reports are also especially necessary for mainstreamed adolescents with ASD, because parents and teachers are less likely to be aware of certain social experiences, especially negative ones (Nishina & Bellmore, 2010), given that there is less adult supervision in more inclusive settings. In research involving both

TD adolescents and adolescents with ASD, it is self-reports of social experiences that are predictive of negative outcomes (Adams & Cantin, 2013; Juvonen et al., 2001; Whitehouse, Durkin, Jaquet, & Ziatas, 2009). Findings from our study (Adams et al., 2014) also support this idea; we found that self-reports of peer victimization had the strongest associations with a latent construct of internalizing symptoms created from both self-report and parent report (βs ranged from 0.50 to 0.68, *ps* < 0.01), and this association held even after controlling for parent reports of peer victimization (βs ranged from 0.46 to 0.75, *ps* < 0.001). Thus, our and others' findings point to the importance of understanding the perspective of the adolescent that is captured by self-reports especially when examining outcomes in adolescents with ASD. There are some issues that must be considered, though, before embracing such measures.

We define peer victimization as being the target, directly or indirectly, of an action/behavior that is intended to harm the target of that action/behavior. Thus, our definition of peer victimization is focused on the perception of the reporter in respect to the intent to harm. This distinction is especially cogent for measuring peer victimization with self-report measures in individuals with ASD given the variability in this group in terms of social cognition (e.g., social perceptions). For example, if an adolescent with ASD reports that no peer victimization has occurred, is this due to not understanding/recognizing that they have actually been targeted for peer victimization, or are they correctly perceiving that no peer victimization has occurred. The groundwork for understanding when and under what circumstances youth with ASD can provide valid reports about their negative peer experiences has not yet been laid. Given the importance of self-reports of these experiences for predicting future outcomes, it is critical for research studies to establish the validity of these measures.

Evidence from our research suggests that adolescents with ASD with higher cognitive and language abilities can indeed provide reliable and valid self-reports of peer victimization, especially for verbal victimization (Adams et al., 2014). In a study of 54 adolescents with ASD spending the majority of their day in a general education setting, we found high internal consistency across the items for verbal peer victimization. In addition, self-reports of verbal peer victimization were correlated with parent reports of verbal victimization, and demonstrated associations with other variables similar to those reported in previous studies with TD adolescents (e.g., internalizing symptoms).

Additionally, study staff assisted all participants as they completed the self-report measures. While participants had no difficulty completing items about verbal or physical victimization, there were some difficulties observed with items about relational victimization. Some adolescents expressed concerns about completing items that asked about events that happened when they were not present (e.g., How do I know someone is talking about me if I am not there?). Even though such questions were raised, the internal consistency across the relational victimization items was adequate and the construct was associated with other variables shown to be correlated with peer victimization in previous studies of typical adolescents. On the other hand, self-reports of relational victimization were not correlated with parent reports of relational victimization. The low correspondence with parent reports may be due to the difficulty of some adolescents to report about those forms of relational aggression that they do not directly witness.

Though adolescents did not report having difficulty understanding the items on the physical victimization scale, the internal consistency across the items on this scale was low. Physical victimization often has lower internal reliability even in self-reports of TD adolescents, which may be due to (1) there being fewer items for this scale (i.e., two items) and (2) physical victimization happens very infrequently.

Together, these findings suggest that there should be more confidence in interpreting findings related to adolescent reports of verbal victimization than relational or physical victimization. Although this does not necessarily mean that adolescents with ASD do not have the ability to provide self-reports about relational or physical victimization, future research is needed to (1) replicate the above findings, (2) identify subgroups of individuals within this group that might be better or worse at providing self-reports; and (3) do more to understand ways to modify current self-report measures to better meet the needs of this group.

In terms of modifying measures of physical victimization, it seems that the low rates of this form of peer victimization might explain the low internal reliability. Specifically, most participants reported that no physical victimization occurred on the two items in our measure, reducing the ability to find consistency across items. Some studies suggest that it might be helpful to consider whether behaviors listed in our current scales (i.e., hit, kick, punch, push, and shove) need to be expanded to capture a fuller range of types of physical aggression directed at those with ASD. For example, Fisher and Taylor (2016) conducted qualitative analysis on answers given by youth with ASD to questions about bullying on the Autism Diagnostic

Observation Schedule (ADOS). They found that most examples of physical victimization described by youth with ASD—such as being poked or having one's shoes tied together—were not behaviors that are typically queried in questionnaires on peer victimization. Yet, these behaviors were identified as salient and distressing by the youth.

In terms of measuring relational peer victimization with self-reports, we may need to think about focusing on aspects of relational aggression that do not require the participant to report about things outside of his/her own point of view. If we look at measures of other forms of peer victimization, items inquire about behaviors clearly directed at the target (e.g., called me names, hit or kicked me), and it seems that many adolescents with ASD are able to report about such behaviors. Thus, we might want to focus on examples of relational aggression that are more apparent, such as actively excluding them from groups or friendships, or trying to turn friends and others against them, rather than on issues such as talking about them when they are not around or spreading rumors or gossip. In addition, as has been shown in research on TD adolescents (Card, Stucky, Sawalani, & Little, 2008), it might be helpful to distinguish between direct (i.e., behaviors directed at the target such as saying "don't play with Tom" when Tom is present) and indirect (i.e., behaviors not directed at the target or when the target is not present, such as saying "don't play with Tom" when Tom is not present) forms of relational peer victimization in adolescents with ASD.

Other issues to keep in mind when using self-reports include findings that self-reports and parent reports of social experiences are often not highly correlated. However, parent report and self-reports of adolescent experiences have each been found to have different degrees of predictive validity when it comes to psychopathology (Achenbach, McConaughy, & Howell, 1987), indicating that the low concordance between self-reports with other reporters should not always be interpreted as an indicator that adolescent self-reports are not valid. Rather, we should strive to ascertain multiple reports of experiences. Since each reporter has his/her own separate insights (as well as shared insights) in reports of experiences, using multiple reporters can provide additional predictive variance in outcome measures. In other words, using multiple reporters provides a more complete picture of experiences, which could also improve our ability to understand the outcome of these experiences.

Additionally, using multiple reporters can help address concerns about shared method variance in cross-sectional survey studies (see below). Finally, using multiple reporters could be especially helpful for those adolescents that may not be as insightful into their own negative peer experiences, and additionally help to understand why rates of parent-reported peer victimization are so much higher than self-reports of peer victimization (Hawker & Boulton, 2000). Further, having multiple reporters, especially a reporter other than self or parent (e.g., teacher, peers, friend), would help to provide reports of experiences outside the purview of parents, who are often not present during peer interactions that take place during adolescence.

3.2 Peer Victimization Versus Bullying

When it comes to issues of measurement and nomenclature, it is important to distinguish between the terms "peer victimization" and "bullying." Often these two terms are used interchangeably, but when it comes to this field of study, not carefully distinguishing between them could negatively affect the findings from studies and confuse conversations about this topic. By definition, bullying is similar to peer victimization in that it involves being a target of aggression, but it differs in that bullying requires that the aggressor to have power over the target of the aggression (Olweus, 1994). This power can manifest in social status, physical size or strength, or psychological control. Thus, all bullying falls under the definition of peer victimization but not all peer victimization falls under the definition of bullying, because there are some instances of peer victimization where the aggressor may not have power over the target.

Bullying can also be interpreted differently by individuals completing surveys. In measuring peer victimization it is important to use items that describe specific behaviors (e.g., hit, kick, call me mean names, etc.), rather than broad terms such as teasing or being mean or bullying. Because these terms lack specificity, they are often defined differently across individuals. For instance, some see the term teasing as when someone, such as a friend, kids them in a friendly manner, while others might see the term teasing as indicating more harmful behavior. The variability in how individuals interpret these terms leads to low reliability in measurement, which directly impacts effect sizes and power in a study. In other words, using such broad terms not only paints a murky picture of the social world, but also makes it more difficult to understand the predictors and outcomes of negative peer experiences, which limits the ability to create effective interventions to address these issues (e.g., Fisher & Taylor, 2016).

The bully/peer victimization distinction is just as important when studying aggression perpetrated by an individual with ASD. It is very important to distinguish aggression from bullying. Using the term bully is potentially problematic when used in the context of individuals with ASD because, as mentioned above, a bully must have a power differential over their victim. It is not so easy to understand how this might work with those with ASD, especially those in a mainstream educational setting. It is more likely the case that an adolescent with ASD might be aggressive without truly having power over his/her victim. While no study of individuals with ASD has teased apart this subtle but important distinction between bullying and being aggressive, it is important to do so because we know from research with TD adolescents that the etiology, forms of aggression, and outcome are very different for those that are aggressive and also victimized compared to those who are aggressive and not victimized. For instance, compared to aggressive nonvictims, aggressive victims are ineffectual and reactive in their aggression, disliked by the peer group, and have high rates of internalizing problems (Adams, Bartlett, & Bukowski, 2010; Perry, Perry, & Kennedy, 1992; Prinstein & Cillessen, 2003; Schwartz, 2000; Schwartz, Proctor, & Chien, 2001). Until we know otherwise, the term bully-victim most likely is not the best term to use with this population, since those with ASD would rarely meet the definition of being a bully.

3.3 Single-Item Measures

Another common measurement issue for studies on this topic concerns utilizing a single item to measure a negative peer experience. Such single-item measures are most likely used in studies of peer experiences of those with ASD because many of the commonly used ASD symptom measures have single items concerning such experiences. Since most studies of adolescents with ASD utilize one or more of these symptom measures, data from many studies designed to test questions on a different topic other than peers are also used to test questions concerning peer experiences. While it has been shown that single-item measures do not always result in increased measurement error (Diamantopoulos, Sarstedt, Fuchs, Wilczynski, & Kaiser, 2012), the nature of constructs that are examined in the study of negative peer experiences make it difficult for single items to effectively measure them. In general, the problem is due to issues discussed above with using the term bullying or teasing, in that single items of these constructs cannot clearly define the construct, nor cover a broad range of experiences that fall under the specific construct. In our own experiences with conducting research in this area, single-item measures of peer victimization (e.g., has your child been bullied or is your child teased?) resulted in null effects or very small effects in comparison to studies that were able to utilize multi-item measures of specific forms of peer victimization. Thus, while using these single items seems advantageous, in that they allow secondary data analyses examining negative social experiences, they are prone to misleading findings that are difficult to replicate across studies.

4. USING AN OBESE COMPARISON GROUP TO PROVIDE EVIDENCE OF THE IMPACT OF PEER VICTIMIZATION ON ADOLESCENTS WITH AUTISM SPECTRUM DISORDER

Those of us working in the field of ASD know and see the devastating impact of negative peer experiences on the lives of adolescents with this diagnosis. Unfortunately, the small number of studies of such experiences and lack of evidence for the ensuing fallout from these experiences have stalled progress in this area.

A particularly significant problem is that we lack the information needed to build empirically informed interventions directed at negative peer experiences targeting those with ASD. For example, because the initial step of linking specific negative experiences to specific outcomes has still not been accomplished, it is not clear which experiences to prioritize in interventions for this group. Currently, most of the empirical evidence on negative peer experiences in adolescents with ASD is provided through a handful of studies that mostly examine the frequency of peer victimization, with very few that test associations with possible outcomes. Testing these associations is needed to understand how adolescents with ASD are affected by specific types of negative experiences, and if/how their experiences are different than other groups.

Often the impact of peer victimization is examined by comparing rates and outcomes of peer victimization to a comparison group. However, the impact of peer victimization on the comparison groups used in many studies of those with ASD is not clear. For one set of comparison groups, adolescents with other developmental disabilities, studies examining the impact of peer victimization are often very limited in terms of methodology and in number (i.e., there are a small number of studies that are cross-sectional with few studies actually testing the outcomes of these negative experiences). For another common comparison group, TD adolescents, a number of longitudinal studies have found that the predictive effects of peer victimization on health and well-being are consistently found to be small (see Reijntjes et al., (2010) meta-analysis). When it is not clear how the comparison group is actually affected by negative experiences, or if the impact is small, it is difficult to interpret the relative impact of peer victimization on those with ASD. Thus, one approach to understanding the effects of peer victimization on the lives of adolescents with ASD might be to place their experiences in contrast to another group for whom the significant impact of peer victimization is well established.

Obese adolescents are one group for whom there is a sizable body of evidence of high rates of peer victimization and strong associations between peer victimization and depressive symptoms. A meta-analysis of 16 studies with over 52,000 participants combined across the studies found obese adolescents were significantly more likely to experience peer victimization than their normal-weighted peers (van Geel, Vedder, & Tanilon, 2014). Additionally, a study using a large scale, nationally representative sample of over 1200 Canadian adolescents found that peer victimization predicted increases in depressive symptoms from ages 12–13 to ages 16–17 in obese adolescents (Adams & Bukowski, 2008). In this study, the standardized effects for predicting these increases in depressive symptoms over the 4 years was between 0.35 and 0.45 for the obese adolescents, which was much larger than the nonsignificant effects (between 0.08 and 0.09) for the non-obese group. The effects for the obese group are also larger than what was seen in a meta-analysis of studies of the general population for the same longitudinal predictive association between peer victimization and depressive symptoms ($r = 0.18$ (95% CI, $0.12 < r < 0.24$), $Z = 6.16$, $P < .001$) (Reijntjes et al., 2010).

These findings for obese adolescents suggest that they would be a particularly helpful group to use as a comparison for adolescents with ASD. Thus, we utilized two separate sets of data, a sample of "high functioning" adolescents with ASD and a group of obese adolescents (see Adams et al., 2014; Adams et al., 2016) to conduct new analyses to examine such comparisons. Specifically, we tested differences between these two groups on rates of different forms of peer victimization, as well as the associations between peer victimization and depressive symptoms. Contrasting the ASD group to the obese group, a group where the impact of peer victimization is clear, will place the findings from the ASD group in a larger context for understanding the impact of peer victimization on those with ASD.

4.1 Methods

All participants were recruited from a large children's hospital in the Midwest United States for two separate studies that used nearly identical methods. For the ASD group, 54 adolescent boys (age $M = 14.6$, $SD = 2.24$, 10.39–17.99 years) were recruited from existing research or clinical registries. Each had previously undergone a comprehensive assessment through either a specialty diagnostic clinic in the Division of Developmental and Behavioral Pediatrics or an ASD-focused research project within a large pediatric hospital. Diagnoses were made by a developmental pediatrician or a clinical psychologist using parent interviews and questionnaires, cognitive and language testing, and the ADOS. All participants with ASD had a previous diagnosis of an ASD, including autism, Asperger's Disorder, or PDD-NOS; were English-speaking; had fluent language abilities, which was defined as using complex sentences on a daily basis; and were between the ages of 10 and 17. The sample was primarily Caucasian (92.6%). See Adams et al. (2014) for additional details concerning recruitment, incentives, and other details of this data collection.

The obese adolescent boy sample was taken from a larger sample of 180 obese adolescents (121 females, 59 males) recruited from a clinic that focused on addressing the needs of obese adolescents. The current analyses included the 59 boys from this group to make it equivalent to the ASD group. The mean age of the sample was 12.78 years ($SD = 1.73$; range: 10–16) and the sample was ethnically diverse (56% African–American, 38% Caucasian, and 6% listed another (i.e., American Indian, Asian, Arabic, Hispanic, or more than one race) or no ethnicity. For the obese group, height and weight were obtained from patient medical records. Using this information, body mass index (BMI) was calculated using the Centers for Disease Control (CDC) growth charts that account for gender and age. Adolescents were defined as obese when their BMIs were equal to or greater than the 95th percentile based on their gender and age. The average BMI for the group of adolescent boys ($M = 34.25$, $SD = 6.7$) was quite high—well above the 97th percentile on the CDC growth chart for boys in this age range. See Adams et al. (2016) for additional details concerning recruitment, incentives, and other details of this data collection.

For both samples, all measures reported below were completed by the adolescents with a member of the study staff present to provide support. The current analyses only examined measures that both samples completed—peer victimization and depressive symptoms. A modified version of the Schwartz Peer Victimization Scale (Schwartz, Farver, Chang, & Lee-Shin, 2002) was utilized to measure several types of self-reported *peer victimization*. For 12 items, adolescents indicated how often they had experienced each type of victimization using a seven-point scale

(1 = "Never happens to me," 2 = "Happens to me once a year," 3 = "Happens to me 2 to 3 times a year," 4 = "Happens to me 4 to 6 times a year," 5 = "Happens to me once or twice a month," 6 = "Happens to me once or twice a week," 7 = "Happens to me almost every day"). The total peer victimization scale score and three subscales scores were used: verbal (e.g., "How often do other kids call you names that hurt your feelings?"), relational (e.g., "How often do other kids gossip or say mean things about you?"), physical (e.g., "How often do other kids hit or push you?"). Scales were created by summing and averaging scores for completed items for each subscale. For the ASD sample all scales had acceptable internal reliability (verbal $\alpha = 0.84$, relational $\alpha = 0.78$; total $\alpha = 0.81$) except physical ($\alpha = 0.55$). For the obese sample, all four scales had acceptable levels of reliability (verbal $\alpha = 0.79$, relational $\alpha = 0.83$, physical $\alpha = 0.81$; total $\alpha = 0.83$). Two additional peer victimization scores were created to measure how often any peer victimization occurred. The first additional score measured if any form of victimization was reported as occurring at least once a week. Victimization was recorded as *occurring at least once a week* if any of the 12 items had a score of 6 or more (i.e., 1 = at least one item was indicated where victimization occurred at least once a week and 0 = no items were indicated where victimization occurred at least once a week). Additionally, victimization was recorded as *happening almost every day* if any of the 12 items had a score of 7 (i.e., 1 = at least one item was indicated where victimization occurred almost every day and 0 = no items were indicated where victimization occurred almost every day).

The Children's Depression Inventory (Kovacs, 1992), a 27-item self-report measure, was utilized to assess cognitive and behavioral *symptoms of depression*. Due to the sensitive nature of the topic, the item pertaining to suicide was omitted from the present study. For each of the remaining 26 items, participants were asked to indicate which statement best described their symptoms over the past 2 weeks with possible scores of 0, 1, or 2. The 26 items were averaged to create a depression score for each participant. The scale had good internal consistency for both groups (ASD $\alpha = 0.88$, obese $\alpha = 0.91$).

4.2 Results/Discussion

Since preliminary analyses found differences in age between the two groups ($t = 5.97$, $P < .01$; ASD $M = 14.61$, $SD = 2.2$; Obese $M = 12.38$, $SD = 1.7$), age was controlled in all analyses described below. To test differences between the two groups on the rates of each of the three types of peer victimization and total rates of peer victimization, four ANCOVAs were conducted with group status as the predictor, one of the peer victimization scores as the outcome, and age as the covariate. As seen in Table 1, there were no significant differences between the groups for any of the types of peer victimization or total peer victimization, with very small effect sizes (i.e., eta squared). Differences between the groups were also tested for the overall frequency of any type of peer victimization occurring in two time periods, at least once or twice a week or almost every day. This provided easily interpretable information about how frequently participants were targeted for these experiences. As seen in Table 1, around 40% of both ASD and obese participants reported experiencing at least one type of peer victimization at least once a week with no significant difference between the two groups. The percentage of those experiencing peer victimization at least once a week is quite large for both groups, especially when compared to a large study of adolescents in the general population that found approximately 10% of participants experienced peer victimization at least once a week (Nansel et al., 2001). When examining those that reported experiencing any type of peer victimization almost every day, the ASD group reported significantly higher rates than the obese group ($X^2 = 3.75$, $P < .05$). More than a third of individuals in the ASD group experienced peer victimization almost every day, a rate that was almost twice as high as the obese group. Given the evidence from multiple studies with large sample sizes indicating that obese adolescents are targeted at higher rates than the general population, these findings

Table 1 Means, Standard Deviations, and Frequency of Peer Victimization in Obese Adolescents and Adolescents With Autism Spectrum Disorder (ASD)

	ASD ($n = 54$)		**Obese ($n = 58$)**			
Victimization Type	***M***	***SD***	***M***	***SD***	***F*-value**	**ES**
Verbal	2.82	1.8	3.07	1.9	0.14	0.00
Relational	3.03	2.1	2.52	1.9	1.47	0.01
Physical	1.89	1.0	2.10	1.7	0.83	0.01
Total	2.66	1.4	2.58	1.7	0.05	0.00
Frequency of Any Type of Victimization	**%(*n*)**		**%(*n*)**			**X^2**
Once/twice a week	46.3(25)		43.1(25)			0.12
Almost every day	35.2(19)		19.0(11)			3.75*

ES, eta squared. **P* < .05, ***P* < .01, ****P* < .001.

of even higher rates of peer victimization in adolescents with ASD are particularly alarming.

Next, we tested the associations between peer victimization and depressive symptoms using partial correlations between each type of peer victimization and depressive symptoms separately for each group, while controlling for age (see Table 2). The first thing that stands out is the relatively large effect sizes for these correlations for both groups. With the exception of physical victimization, all the correlations are larger than 0.50. Hawker and Boulton's (2000) meta-analysis testing the associations between measures of total peer victimization and various types of psychological adjustment in TD populations (using similar methods) found the average correlation between total victimization and depressive symptoms across nine studies to be 0.45, which is smaller than the correlations found for our ASD and obese samples (0.68 and 0.55, respectively). While the correlations in the meta-analysis and those in our studies cannot be directly compared, we provide the average correlation across these meta-analysis studies to help put the correlations in our studies in perspective, especially since the studies in the meta-analysis and our studies are the same design (i.e., cross-sectional and do not control for possible issues of shared method variance). Previous studies have directly tested the differences between these effects and found that the longitudinal effects of peer victimization on internalizing symptoms was significantly stronger in obese adolescents than nonobese adolescents (Adams & Bukowski, 2008; Adams & Cantin, 2013). Together these findings suggest that the effects of peer victimization on depressive symptoms are stronger in these two at-risk groups than what we see in typical samples.

Table 2 Partial Correlations Between Various Forms of Peer Victimization and Depressive Symptoms in Adolescents With Autism Spectrum Disorder (ASD) and Obese Adolescents

	Partial Correlation Between Victimization and the CDI	
Type of Victimization	**ASD**	**Obese**
Verbal	0.66***	0.52***
Relational	0.57***	0.51***
Physical	0.32*	0.48***
Total	0.68***	0.55***

Partial correlations control for age. *$P < .05$, **$P < .01$, ***$P < .001$; *CDI*, Children's Depression Inventory.

Multiple regression analyses tested for differences between the two groups in the associations between each of the types of peer victimization and depressive symptoms by testing the group by peer victimization interaction in each analysis. For each regression, age (i.e., control variable), a centered peer victimization measure (i.e., predictor variable), and the group measure (i.e., moderator, ASD vs. obese) were entered on the first step. On the second step, the interaction terms between peer victimization and group was entered. No significant interactions were found (all $\Delta R^2 < 0.004$, all $ps > 0.43$) indicating no significant differences between the groups for the associations between the peer victimization and depressive symptoms.

To provide additional evidence of the association between peer victimization and depressive symptoms, we tested the differences between the groups based on frequency of peer victimization (i.e., Once/twice a week vs. not; Almost every day vs. not) on depressive symptoms using independent sample *t*-tests. As seen in Table 3, there were significant differences with large effect sizes in rates of depressive symptoms between those who reported frequently experiencing peer victimization and those who did not for both the ASD and the obese samples and similar to the results of the partial correlation analyses, the effect sizes of these differences between these groups on depressive symptoms were large. ANOVAs found no significant differences for the interaction between the sample groups and the peer victimization frequency groups on the depressive symptoms measure, suggesting there were no significant differences between the ASD and obese samples for the effects of the victimization groups on depressive symptoms.

Table 3 Differences in Depressive Symptoms Between Those Who Experience Peer Victimization Often and Those Who Do Not Experience Peer Victimization Often in Adolescents With Autism Spectrum Disorder (ASD) and Obese Adolescents

	M(SD)			
Group	**No**	**Yes**	**t-test**	**Cohen's *d***
Victimized Once/Twice a Week				
ASD	0.165(0.15)	0.550(0.26)	5.43***	1.36
Obese	0.261(0.23)	0.543(0.36)	3.66***	0.93
Victimized Almost Every Day				
ASD	0.219(0.21)	0.570(0.26)	5.44***	1.28
Obese	0.301(0.25)	0.731(0.36)	4.66***	1.38

*$P < .05$, **$P < .01$, ***$P < .001$.

Overall these findings provide preliminary evidence that the negative impact of peer victimization on the lives of adolescents with ASD is similar to, and in a few instances more so, than for obese adolescents, a group where the relatively high rates of peer victimization and the impact of peer victimization on depressive symptoms are well-documented. Both groups were found to commonly experience various types of peer victimization, with verbal victimization occurring most frequently. Unfortunately, more than a third of the adolescents with ASD reported experiencing some form of peer victimization almost every day, a rate almost double that found in the obese group. These rates are especially concerning given the strong associations of peer victimization with depressive symptoms in this study. Specifically, the absolute sizes of effects between the various measurements of peer victimization and depressive symptoms were large with some instances of effect sizes being well over 1 *SD*.

Overall, these findings provide important insights in terms of the impact that peer victimization has on the mental health of adolescents with ASD. To move this field forward, longitudinal studies that collect data from adolescents with ASD are sorely needed, not only to disentangle the directionality of the links between peer victimization and depressive symptoms, but also to understand how negative peer experiences change over time in this high-risk group.

5. ISSUES TO CONSIDER IN FUTURE STUDIES OF NEGATIVE PEER EXPERIENCES IN ADOLESCENTS WITH AUTISM SPECTRUM DISORDER

5.1 Incorporating Typically Developing Peers

We think it is important for studies and interventions to explore ways that TD peers may serve as an additional resource for combatting the negative peer experiences of adolescents with ASD. While interventions have been shown to improve some symptoms of ASD, the majority of individuals with ASD continue to exhibit some degree of social deficits throughout their lives (Anderson, Liang, & Lord, 2014; Shattuck et al., 2007). Additionally, the multiple types of social deficits that individual with ASD face would make it difficult for interventions targeting peer experiences to be able to successfully address all the various skills and strategies required to effectively reduce all types of peer problems that they may face. In our own experiences developing programs to address peer victimization in this group, we have found that strategies found to be successful in interventions targeting TD adolescents are not always easily transferable to those with ASD.

In light of these challenges, interventions to reduce peer victimization among individuals with ASD must consider targeting TD peers. In fact, the most successful antipeer victimization interventions for TD adolescents involve targeting the larger peer group to promote directly and indirectly intervening, not reinforcing aggressive actions, and creating positive peer cultures (Kärnä et al., 2013, A. Kärnä, M. Voeten, T. D. Little, E. Poskiparta, E. Alanen et al., 2011, A. Kärnä, M. Voeten, T. D. Little, E. Poskiparta, A. Kaljonen, et al., 2011). However, successful interventions that target peers cannot be utilized in their current form, as they need to be modified around the issues that are unique to adolescents with ASD. For instance, previous studies have found that for peers to successfully intervene, there is a need to create empathy and positive feeling toward those being victimized. This can be difficult for targeted individuals with ASD since many behaviors that this group exhibit can lead to negative perceptions, attributions, and dislike (see above).

Due to TD peers' lack of understanding about ASD in general, they are more likely to interpret the behaviors that individuals in this group exhibit in a negative manner. This lack of understanding may result in peers incorrectly attributing the causes of these behaviors as being internal to the individual (Graham & Juvonen, 2001). Attribution theory tells us that these sorts of attributions (i.e., internal and controllable) lead to negative evaluations and dislike of the individual exhibiting such behaviors. Indeed, as mentioned previously, typical peers express more negative and less positive descriptions of individuals with ASD (Bauminger & Kasari, 2000; Chamberlain et al., 2007; Humphrey & Symes, 2010, 2011; Jones & Frederickson, 2010; Locke et al., 2010; Lyons et al., 2011; Petrina et al., 2014). It is difficult, then, to ask peers to intervene when negative peer experiences are happening to those with ASD, given that they may have negative feelings about the person with ASD or even feel that the person brought these experiences onto themselves. Thus, interventions that attempt to involve TD peers must first educate peers about ASD in general, the types of behaviors characteristic of ASD, and how these behaviors are symptoms of their disorder and as such, are not easily controllable for those with ASD. Further, even if the TD peers do not have negative attributions about an individual with ASD, they might be hesitant to reach out to intervene because they do not know the best way to interact or help a peer with ASD.

When looking for ways get peers involved in helping to protect those with ASD from negative peer experiences, it is important to not only address the negative attributions and feelings they might have toward an individual with ASD but also explain how to support and protect individuals in this group. Research in TD adolescents has shown that perpetrators of peer victimization are less likely to target individuals who are viewed positively by the peer group. Potential aggressors know that their aggression toward that individual would result in negative consequences from the peer group or would not have a positive impact on the social status they might be trying to attain through bullying. The field must study and develop ways to educate TD peers to promote positive interactions with their peers with ASD.

5.2 Gender

Gender differences in peer experiences are common in studies of TD adolescents. Significant gender differences are apparent in TD adolescent friendships, in terms of activities, time spent, and characteristics (Rose & Rudolph, 2006), as well as in peer victimization (e.g., rates of different types and content of victimization; Hong & Espelage, 2012). As mentioned above, studies of TD adolescents have found that males and females often experience different forms of bullying, with boys experiencing more physical bullying (Carbone-Lopez, Esbensen, & Brick, 2010), girls experiencing more relational forms (Murray-Close, Ostrov, & Crick, 2007), and boys and girls experiencing similar levels of verbal bullying but with topics of verbal bullying differing by gender (Duncan, 1999; Gruber & Fineran, 2008). Because social experiences often vary as a function of gender, it is clear that successful interventions targeting social experience must take gender into account. For example, antipeer victimization curricula for adolescent girls account for the fact that, while boys and girls are equally likely to experience direct verbal bullying, the content of verbal attacks directed at girls are more likely to be of a sexual nature or to concern appearance (Duncan, 1999; Gruber & Fineran, 2008). Thus interventions need to incorporate this issue into the strategies to address these specific forms of verbal bullying to ensure that the participants are able to recognize, identify, and utilize the strategies.

Despite its importance in this area of research, gender is seldom given proper attention as a variable in studies of ASD (Halladay et al., 2015). While it can be difficult to ascertain large numbers of girls for these studies because the sex ratio is higher for boys (4 or 5 to 1; Lai, Lombardo, Auyeung,

Chakrabarti, & Baron-Cohen, 2015), it is essential to consider the issue of gender in studies of social or peer relations. In fact, outside of the ASD realm, it would be unheard of to analyze boys and girls together in a study of adolescent social experiences.

5.3 Internalizing Problems and Negative Peer Experiences

Adolescents with ASD are at particular risk for internalizing problems. Lifetime estimates of internalizing disorders are as high as 52% for depression and 65% for anxiety disorders, compared to rates of 5% and 20% reported in TD adolescents (E. J. Costello, H. Egger, & A. Angold, 2005; E. J. Costello, H. L. Egger, & A. Angold, 2005; Lever & Geurts, 2016; Leyfer et al., 2006; van Steensel, Bogels & Perrin, 2011). Rates of internalizing problems increase during adolescence/young adulthood for people with ASD (Gotham, Bishop, Brunwasser, & Lord, 2014), resulting in an overall diminished quality of life for this group (Hong, Bishop-Fitzpatrick, Smith, Greenberg, & Mailick, 2016; Leyfer et al., 2006; Mayes, Gorman, Hillwig-Garcia, & Syed, 2013; Taylor & Gotham, 2016; van Steensel et al., 2011). This issue is so impactful that for many, otherwise verbally and cognitively capable youth with ASD seeking treatment, the primary treatment goals focus on internalizing symptoms rather than ASD symptoms per se (Kerns & Kendall, 2012). Failing to effectively understand and treat internalizing disorders has grave consequences with recent studies finding staggering rates of suicide attempts and completions among adults with ASD (Cassidy et al., 2014; Hirvikoski et al., 2016; Mukaddes & Fateh, 2010; Segers & Rawana, 2014).

The substantial risk of both negative peer experiences and internalizing problems among individuals with ASD is additionally concerning because such experiences are shown to be predictive of increasing internalizing symptoms over time in TD and obese adolescents (Adams & Bukowski, 2008; Adams & Cantin, 2013; Reijntjes et al., 2010). Cross-sectional studies have found similar concurrent associations in those with ASD (Adams et al., 2014; Rosbrook & Whittingham, 2010; Storch et al., 2012). This suggests that interventions that target internalizing symptoms in this group may need to also address negative peer experiences. Currently most treatment protocols for internalizing problems that have been developed for use with individuals with ASD (Dove et al., 2012; Nadeau et al., 2011; Reaven, Blakeley-Smith, Culhane-Shelburne, & Hepburn, 2012; Storch et al., 2015; Wood et al., 2015) primarily target biological (e.g., through selective serotonin reuptake inhibitors) and cognitive (e.g., through cognitive behavioral therapy) factors known to underlie internalizing problems. Available treatments often ignore the experiential factors that may precipitate internalizing symptoms, even though it is well known that biological, cognitive, and experiential factors operate separately and in conjunction with one another to increase risk for internalizing problems (Eley et al., 2004; Garcia-Toro & Aguirre, 2007; Hankin & Abramson, 2001; Hicks, DiRago, Iacono, & McGue, 2009; Lonsdorf et al., 2009). If these internalizing symptoms do arise as a result of negative experiences that occur almost daily or weekly for many in this group, interventions that target only dysfunctional thought processes or neurotransmitters are unlikely to yield significant and lasting benefits. Thus, there seems to be an imperative to incorporate antinegative peer experience strategies into treatment plans for addressing internalizing symptoms in adolescents with ASD.

The absence of such strategies in current treatment plans is most likely due to gaps in our understanding of how internalizing issues are precipitated by negative experiences in adolescents with ASD. Here we will talk about two barriers with each barrier being multifaceted. The first barrier is that few studies of negative peer experiences in this group actually test the associations with outcomes such as internalizing symptoms, and almost all studies that do test this association are cross-sectional. This means that we do not have direct evidence that negative peer experiences actually predict increases in internalizing symptoms in adolescents with ASD. Additionally, the lack of longitudinal studies on this topic also means that we do not know the developmental trajectories of these experiences. We therefore lack information about the ideal developmental window for targeting these experiences in this group.

The second barrier is identifying the specific types of experiences that precipitate internalizing symptoms. There are multiple problems to be addressed in this respect. One, most individuals with ASD are dealing with multiple negative types of experiences due to the various issues outlined above. Two, due to deficits in social cognitions and communication, we cannot assume that all types of experiences that TD individuals deem to be negative have the same effects on those with ASD. These two issues mean that we must first identify what experiences are predictive of internalizing problems in this group to be able to know what experiences should be addressed in treatment. Once specific experiences are identified, current options for combatting internalizing problems in ASD can be expanded. For example, interventions can be created to deter negative experiences that predict increasing internalizing symptoms, and existing interventions will also benefit from the new information gained by modifying the intervention to target those specific experiences that are most important to mental health. For example, if we find that verbal peer victimization has a strong predictive association with internalizing problems and no associations are found in other interactions involving close personal interactions, then social skills interventions could be modified to target the specific skills that address verbal peer victimization, rather than focusing on teaching the very different set of skills required for other experiences that involve close interpersonal interactions.

6. CONCLUSION

In conclusion, the last decade has seen a major increase in studies of peer victimization in ASD, but numerous questions remain. While accumulating evidence suggests that adolescents with ASD experience very high rates of peer victimization, and studies indicate significant associations between peer victimization and internalizing problems in this group, there is a clear need for high quality, longitudinal studies to delineate which forms of peer victimization have the greatest effects for whom, and more importantly, what can be done to prevent or minimize the negative effects of these experiences. Strategies that will be important to incorporate in these studies include the use of well validated measures of peer victimization that consider different types of peer victimization, ascertaining reports from multiple informants (including self-report when appropriate), identifying appropriate comparison groups to evaluate against those with ASD, and carefully considering relevant phenotypic variables in the ASD groups (e.g., sex, cognitive ability, profiles of social strengths and difficulties). As interventions are being developed and validated, it will be important to look beyond strategies that directly target the adolescents with ASD, and explore how the larger peer group might be recruited to reduce negative peer experiences for individuals with ASD.

REFERENCES

Achenbach, T. M., McConaughy, S. H., & Howell, C. T. (1987). Child/adolescent behavioral and emotional problems: Implications of cross-informant correlations for situational specificity. *Psychological Bulletin, 101*(2), 213–232. http://dx.doi.org/10.1037/0033-2909.101.2.213.

Adams, R. E., Bartlett, N. H., & Bukowski, W. M. (2010). Peer victimization and social dominance as intervening variables of the link between peer liking and relational aggression. *The Journal of Early Adolescence, 30*(1), 102–121. http://dx.doi.org/10.1177/0272431609342985.

Adams, R. E., & Bukowski, W. M. (2008). Peer victimization as a predictor of depression and body mass index in obese and non-obese adolescents. *Journal of Child Psychology and Psychiatry, 49*(8), 858–866. http://dx.doi.org/10.1111/j.1469-7610.2008.01886.x.

Adams, R. E., & Cantin, S. (2013). Self-disclosure in friendships as the moderator of the association between peer victimization and depressive symptoms in overweight adolescents. *The Journal of Early Adolescence, 33*(3), 341–362. http://dx.doi.org/10.1177/0272431612441068.

Adams, R. E., Fredstrom, B. K., Duncan, A. W., Holleb, L. J., & Bishop, S. L. (2014). Using self- and parent-reports to test the association between peer victimization and internalizing symptoms in verbally fluent adolescents with ASD. *Journal of Autism and Developmental Disorders, 44*(4), 861–872. http://dx.doi.org/10.1007/s10803-013-1938-0.

Adams, R. E., Fredstrom, B. K., Peets, K. K., Hodges, E. V. E., Bowker, J. C., Holleb, L. J, & Gilman, R. (2016). Validating a measure of friends' responses to self-disclosure in adolescent obese and public school samples. *Journal of Clinical Child and Adolescent Psychology*. http://dx.doi.org/10.1080/15374416.2015.1094738.

Adams, R. E., Santo, J. B., & Bukowski, W. M. (2011). The presence of a best friend buffers the effects of negative experiences. *Developmental Psychology, 47*(6), 1786–1791. http://dx.doi.org/10.1037/a0025401.

Anderson, D. K., Liang, J. W., & Lord, C. (2014). Predicting young adult outcome among more and less cognitively able individuals with autism spectrum disorders. *Journal of Child Psychology and Psychiatry, 55*(5), 485–494.

Bauminger, N., & Kasari, C. (2000). Loneliness and friendship in high-functioning children with autism. *Child Development, 71*(2), 447–456. http://dx.doi.org/10.1111/1467-8624.00156.

Bear, G., Mantz, L. S., Glutting, J. J., Yang, C., & Boyer, D. E. (2015). Differences in bullying victimization between students with and without disabilities. *School Psychology Review, 44*, 98–116.

Bowker, J. C., Adams, R. E., Fredstrom, B. K., & Gilman, R. (2014). Experiences of being ignored by peers during late adolescence: Linkages to psychological maladjustment. *Merrill-Palmer Quarterly, 60*(3), 328–354. http://dx.doi.org/10.13110/merrpalmquar1982.60.3.0328.

Cappadocia, M. C., Weiss, J. A., & Pepler, D. (2012). Bullying experiences among children and youth with autism spectrum disorders. *Journal of Autism and Developmental Disorders, 42*(2), 266–277. http://dx.doi.org/10.1007/s10803-011-1241-x.

Carbone-Lopez, K., Esbensen, F., & Brick, B. T. (2010). Correlates and consequences of peer victimization: Gender differences in direct and indirect forms of bullying. *Youth Violence and Juvenile Justice, 8*(4), 332–350. http://dx.doi.org/10.1177/1541204010362954.

Card, N. A., & Little, T. D. (2006). Proactive and reactive aggression in childhood and adolescence: A meta-analysis of differential relations with psychosocial adjustment. *International Journal of Behavioral Development, 30*(5), 466–480. http://dx.doi.org/10.1177/0165025406071904.

Card, N. A., Stucky, B. D., Sawalani, G. M., & Little, T. D. (2008). Direct and indirect aggression during childhood and adolescence: A meta-analytic review of gender differences, intercorrelations, and relations to maladjustment. *Child Development, 79*(5), 1185–1229. http://dx.doi.org/10.1111/j.1467-8624.2008.01184.x.

Cassidy, S., Bradley, P., Robinson, J., Allison, C., McHugh, M., & Baron-Cohen, S. (2014). Suicidal ideation and suicide plans or attempts in adults with Asperger's syndrome attending a specialist diagnostic clinic: A clinical cohort study. *The Lancet Psychiatry, 1*(2), 142–147. http://dx.doi.org/10.1016/S2215-0366(14)70248-2.

Chamberlain, B., Kasari, C., & Rotheram-Fuller, E. (2007). Involvement or isolation? The social networks of children with autism in regular classrooms. *Journal of Autism and Developmental Disorders, 37*(2), 230–242. http://dx.doi.org/10.1007/s10803-006-0164-4.

Costello, E. J., Egger, H., & Angold, A. (2005). 10-year research update review: The epidemiology of child and adolescent psychiatric disorders: I. Methods and public health burden. *Journal of the American Academy of Child and Adolescent Psychiatry, 44*(10), 972–986. http://dx.doi.org/10.1097/01.chi.0000172552.41596.6f.

Costello, E. J., Egger, H. L., & Angold, A. (2005). The developmental epidemiology of anxiety disorders: Phenomenology, prevalence, and comorbidity. *Child and Adolescent Psychiatric Clinics of North America, 14*(4), 631–648. http://dx.doi.org/10.1016/j.chc.2005.06.003.

Diamantopoulos, A., Sarstedt, M., Fuchs, C., Wilczynski, P., & Kaiser, S. (2012). Guidelines for choosing between multi-item and single-item scales for construct measurement: A predictive validity perspective. *Journal of the Academy of Marketing Science, 40*(3), 434–449. http://dx.doi.org/10.1007/s11747-011-0300-3.

Dove, D., Warren, Z., McPheeters, M. L., Taylor, J. L., Sathe, N. A., & Veenstra-VanderWeele, J. (2012). Medications for adolescents and young adults with autism spectrum disorders: A systematic review. *Pediatrics, 130*(4), 717–726. http://dx.doi.org/10.1542/peds.2012-0683.

Duncan, N. (1999). *Sexual bullying: Gender conflict and pupil culture in secondary schools*. New York, NY: Routledge.

Eley, T. C., Sugden, K., Corsico, A., Gregory, A. M., Sham, P., McGuffin, P., … Craig, I. W. (2004). Gene-environment interaction analysis of serotonin system markers with adolescent depression. *Molecular Psychiatry, 9*(10), 908–915. http://dx.doi.org/10.1038/sj.mp.4001546.

Fisher, M. H., & Taylor, J. L. (2016). Let's talk about it: Peer victimization experiences as reported by adolescents with autism spectrum disorder. *Autism, 20*(4), 402–411. http://dx.doi.org/10.1177/1362361315585948.

Garcia-Toro, M., & Aguirre, I. (2007). Biopsychosocial model in depression revisited. *Medical Hypotheses, 68*(3), 683–691. http://dx.doi.org/10.1016/j.mehy.2006.02.049.

van Geel, M., Vedder, P., & Tanilon, J. (2014). Are overweight and obese youths more often bullied by their peers? A meta-analysis on the correlation between weight status and bullying. *International Journal of Obesity (2005), 38*(10), 1263–1267. http://dx.doi.org/10.1038/ijo.2014.117.

Ghaziuddin, M., Ghaziuddin, N., & Greden, J. (2002). Depression in persons with autism: Implications for research and clinical care. *Journal of Autism and Developmental Disorders, 32*(4), 299–306. http://dx.doi.org/10.1023/a:1016330802348.

Gooren, E. M., van Lier, P. A., Stegge, H., Terwogt, M. M., & Koot, H. M. (2011). The development of conduct problems and depressive symptoms in early elementary school children: The role of peer rejection. *Journal of Clinical Child and Adolescent Psychology, 40*(2), 245–253. http://dx.doi.org/10.1080/15374416.2011.546045.

Gotham, K., Bishop, S. L., Brunwasser, S., & Lord, C. (2014). Rumination and perceived impairment associated with depressive symptoms in a verbal adolescent-adult ASD sample. *Autism research: Official Journal of the International Society for Autism Research*, 7(3), 381–391. http://dx.doi.org/10.1002/aur.1377.

Graham, S., & Juvonen, J. (2001). An attributional approach to peer victimization. In J. S. Graham (Ed.), *Peer harassment in school. The plight of the vulnerable and victimized.* (pp. 49–72). New York: Guilford Press.

Gruber, J. E., & Fineran, S. (2008). Comparing the impact of bullying and sexual harassment victimization on the mental and physical health of adolescents. *Sex Roles, 59*(1–2), 1–13. http://dx.doi.org/10.1007/s11199-008-9431-5.

Halladay, A. K., Bishop, S., Constantino, J. N., Daniels, A. M., Koenig, K., Palmer, K., ... Szatmari, P. (2015). Sex and gender differences in autism spectrum disorder: Summarizing evidence gaps and identifying emerging areas of priority. *Molecular Autism, 6*, 36. http://dx.doi.org/10.1186/s13229-015-0019-y.

Hankin, B. L., & Abramson, L. Y. (2001). Development of gender differences in depression: An elaborated cognitive vulnerability-transactional stress theory. *Psychological Bulletin, 127*(6), 773–796.

Hawker, D. S. J., & Boulton, M. J. (2000). Twenty years' research on peer victimization and psychosocial maladjustment: A meta-analytic review of cross-sectional studies. *Journal of Child Psychology and Psychiatry, 41*(4), 441–455. http://dx.doi.org/10.1111/1469-7610.00629.

Hicks, B. M., DiRago, A. C., Iacono, W. G., & McGue, M. (2009). Gene-environment interplay in internalizing disorders: Consistent findings across six environmental risk factors. *Journal of Child Psychology and Psychiatry and Allied Disciplines, 50*(10), 1309–1317. http://dx.doi.org/10.1111/j.1469-7610.2009.02100.x.

Hirvikoski, T., Mittendorfer-Rutz, E., Boman, M., Larsson, H., Lichtenstein, P., & Bölte, S. (2016). Premature mortality in autism spectrum disorder. *The British Journal of Psychiatry, 208*(3), 232–238. http://dx.doi.org/10.1192/bjp.bp.114.160192.

Hodges, E. V., Malone, M. J., & Perry, D. G. (1997). Individual risk and social risk as interacting determinants of victimization in the peer group. *Developmental Psychology, 33*(6), 1032–1039.

Hodges, E. V. E., Boivin, M., Vitaro, F., & Bukowski, W. M. (1999). The power of friendship: Protection against an escalating cycle of peer victimization. *Developmental Psychology, 35*(1), 94–101. http://dx.doi.org/10.1037/0012-1649.35.1.94.

Hong, J., Bishop-Fitzpatrick, L., Smith, L. E., Greenberg, J. S., & Mailick, M. R. (2016). Factors associated with subjective quality of life of adults with autism spectrum disorder: Self-report versus maternal reports. *Journal of Autism and Developmental Disorders, 46*(4), 1368–1378. http://dx.doi.org/10.1007/s10803-015-2678-0.

Hong, J. S., & Espelage, D. L. (2012). A review of research on bullying and peer victimization in school: An ecological system analysis. *Aggression and Violent Behavior, 17*(4), 311–322. http://dx.doi.org/10.1016/j.avb.2012.03.003.

Humphrey, N., & Symes, W. (2010). Perceptions of social support and experience of bullying among pupils with autistic spectrum disorders in mainstream secondary schools. *European Journal of Special Needs Education, 25*(1), 77–91. http://dx.doi.org/10.1080/08856250903450855.

Humphrey, N., & Symes, W. (2011). Peer interaction patterns among adolescents with autistic spectrum disorders (ASDs) in mainstream school settings. *Autism, 15*(4), 397–419. http://dx.doi.org/10.1177/1362361310387804.

Jones, A. P., & Frederickson, N. (2010). Multi-informant predictors of social inclusion for students with autism spectrum disorders attending mainstream school. *Journal of Autism and Developmental Disorders, 40*(9), 1094–1103. http://dx.doi.org/10.1007/s10803-010-0957-3.

Juvonen, J., Nishina, A., & Graham, S. (2001). Self-views versus peer perceptions of victim status among early adolescents. In J. Juvonen, & S. Graham (Eds.), *Peer harassment in school: The plight of the vulnerable and victimized.* (pp. 105–124). New York, NY, US: Guilford Press.

Kärnä, A., Voeten, M., Little, T. D., Alanen, E., Poskiparta, E., & Salmivalli, C. (2013). Effectiveness of the KiVa antibullying program: Grades 1–3 and 7–9. *Journal of Educational Psychology, 105*(2), 535–551. http://dx.doi.org/10.1037/a0030417.

Kärnä, A., Voeten, M., Little, T. D., Poskiparta, E., Alanen, E., & Salmivalli, C. (2011). Going to scale: A nonrandomized nationwide trial of the KiVa antibullying program for grades 1–9. *Journal of Consulting and Clinical Psychology, 79*(6), 796–805. http://dx.doi.org/10.1037/a0025740.

Kärnä, A., Voeten, M., Little, T. D., Poskiparta, E., Kaljonen, A., & Salmivalli, C. (2011). A large-scale evaluation of the KiVa antibullying program: Grades 4–6. *Child Development, 82*(1), 311–330. http://dx.doi.org/10.111/j.1467-8624.2010.01557.x.

Kerns, C. M., & Kendall, P. C. (2012). The presentation and classification of anxiety in autism spectrum disorder. *Clinical Psychology: Science and Practice, 19*(4), 323–347. http://dx.doi.org/10.1111/cpsp.12009.

Kloosterman, P. H., Kelley, E. A., Craig, W. M., Parker, J. D. A., & Javier, C. (2013). Types and experiences of bullying in adolescents with an autism spectrum disorder. *Research in Autism Spectrum Disorders,* 7(7), 824–832. http://dx.doi.org/10.1016/j.rasd.2013.02.013.

Kovacs, M. (1992). *Children's depression inventory (CDI): Multi-health systems.*

Lai, M. C., Lombardo, M. V., Auyeung, B., Chakrabarti, B., & Baron-Cohen, S. (2015). Sex/gender differences and autism: Setting the scene for future research. *Journal of the American Academy of Child and Adolescent Psychiatry, 54*(1), 11–24. http://dx.doi.org/10.1016/j.jaac.2014.10.003.

Lever, A. G., & Geurts, H. M. (2016). Psychiatric co-occurring symptoms and disorders in young, middle-aged, and older adults with autism spectrum disorder. *Journal of Autism and Developmental Disorders, 46*(6), 1916–1930. http://dx.doi.org/10.1007/s10803-016-2722-8.

Leyfer, O. T., Folstein, S. E., Bacalman, S., Davis, N. O., Dinh, E., Morgan, J., … Lainhart, J. E. (2006). Comorbid psychiatric disorders in children with autism: Interview development and rates of disorders. *Journal of Autism and Developmental Disorders, 36*(7), 849–861. http://dx.doi.org/10.1007/s10803-006-0123-0.

Little, L. (2002). Middle-class mothers' perceptions of peer and sibling victimization among children with Asperger's syndrome and nonverbal learning disorders. *Issues in Comprehensive Pediatric Nursing, 25*(1), 43–57.

Locke, J., Ishijima, E. H., Kasari, C., & London, N. (2010). Loneliness, friendship quality and the social networks of adolescents with high-functioning autism in an inclusive school setting. *Journal of Research in Special Educational Needs, 10*(2), 74–81. http://dx.doi.org/10.1111/j.1471-3802.2010.01148.x.

Lonsdorf, T. B., Weike, A. I., Nikamo, P., Schalling, M., Hamm, A. O., & Ohman, A. (2009). Genetic gating of human fear learning and extinction: Possible implications for gene-environment interaction in anxiety disorder. *Psychological Science, 20*(2), 198–206. http://dx.doi.org/10.1111/j.1467-9280.2009.02280.x.

Lyons, J., Cappadocia, M. C., & Weiss, J. A. (2011). BRIEF report: Social characteristics of students with autism spectrum disorders across classroom settings. *Journal on Developmental Disabilities, 17*(1), 77–82.

Maiano, C., Normand, C. L., Salvas, M. C., Moullec, G., & Aime, A. (2016). Prevalence of school bullying among youth with autism spectrum disorders: A systematic review and meta-analysis. *Autism Research, 9*(6), 601–615. http://dx.doi.org/10.1002/aur.1568.

Mayes, S. D., Gorman, A. A., Hillwig-Garcia, J., & Syed, E. (2013). Suicide ideation and attempts in children with autism. *Research in Autism Spectrum Disorders,* 7(1), 109–119. http://dx.doi.org/10.1016/j.rasd.2012.07.009.

Mukaddes, N. M., & Fateh, R. (2010). High rates of psychiatric co-morbidity in individuals with Asperger's disorder. *World Journal of Biological Psychiatry, 11*(2 Pt 2), 486–492. http://dx.doi.org/10.1080/15622970902789130.

Murray-Close, D., Ostrov, J. M., & Crick, N. R. (2007). A short-term longitudinal study of growth of relational aggression during middle childhood: Associations with gender, friendship intimacy, and internalizing problems. *Development and Psychopathology, 19*(01), 187–203. http://dx.doi.org/10.1017/S0954579407070101.

Nadeau, J., Sulkowski, M. L., Ung, D., Wood, J. J., Lewin, A. B., Murphy, T. K., … Storch, E. A. (2011). Treatment of comorbid anxiety and autism spectrum disorders. *Neuropsychiatry, 1*(6), 567–578.

Nansel, T. R., Overpeck, M., Pilla, R. S., Ruan, W., Simons-Morton, B., & Scheidt, P. (2001). Bullying behaviors among us youth: Prevalence and association with psychosocial adjustment. *JAMA, 285*(16), 2094–2100. http://dx.doi.org/10.1001/jama.285.16.2094.

Nishina, A., & Bellmore, A. (2010). When might peer aggression, victimization, and conflict have its largest impact? Microcontextual considerations. *The Journal of Early Adolescence, 30*(1), 5–26. http://dx.doi.org/10.1177/0272431609350928.

Nowell, K. P., Brewton, C. M., & Goin-Kochel, R. P. (2014). A multi-rater study on being teased among children/adolescents with autism spectrum disorder (ASD) and their typically developing siblings: Associations with ASD symptoms. *Focus on Autism and Other Developmental Disabilities*. http://dx.doi.org/10.1177/1088357614522292.

Olweus, D. (1994). Bullying at school. *Agressive Behavior*, 97–103 (Springer U.S.).

Perry, D. G., Perry, L. C., & Kennedy, E. (1992). Conflict and the development of antisocial behavior. In C. U. Shantz, & W. W. Hartup (Eds.), *Conflict in child and adolescent development* (pp. 301–329). New York: Cambridge University Press.

Petrina, N., Carter, M., & Stephenson, J. (2014). The nature of friendship in children with autism spectrum disorders: A systematic review. *Research in Autism Spectrum Disorders, 8*(2), 111–126. http://dx.doi.org/10.1016/j.rasd.2013.10.016.

Polanin, J. R., Espelage, D. L., & Pigott, T. D. (2012). A meta-analysis of school-based bullying prevention programs' effects on bystander intervention behavior. *School Psychology Review, 41*(1), 47–65.

Prinstein, M. J., Boergers, J., & Vernberg, E. M. (2001). Overt and relational aggression in adolescents: Social-psychological adjustment of aggressors and victims. *Journal of Clinical Child and Adolescent Psychology, 30*(4), 479–491. http://dx.doi.org/10.1207/s15374424jccp3004_05.

Prinstein, M. J., & Cillessen, A. H. N. (2003). Forms and functions of adolescent peer aggression associated with high levels of peer status. *Merrill-Palmer Quarterly, 49*(3), 310–342. http://dx.doi.org/10.1353/mpq.2003.0015.

Reaven, J., Blakeley-Smith, A., Culhane-Shelburne, K., & Hepburn, S. (2012). Group cognitive behavior therapy for children with high-functioning autism spectrum disorders and anxiety: A randomized trial. *Journal of Child Psychology and Psychiatry and Allied Disciplines, 53*(4), 410–419.

Reijntjes, A., Kamphuis, J. H., Prinzie, P., & Telch, M. J. (2010). Peer victimization and internalizing problems in children: A meta-analysis of longitudinal studies. *Child Abuse & Neglect, 34*(4), 244–252. http://dx.doi.org/10.1016/j.chiabu.2009.07.009.

Rosbrook, A., & Whittingham, K. (2010). Autistic traits in the general population: What mediates the link with depressive and anxious symptomatology? *Research in Autism Spectrum Disorders, 4*(3), 415–424. http://dx.doi.org/10.1016/j.rasd.2009.10.012.

Rose, A. J., & Rudolph, K. D. (2006). A review of sex differences in peer relationship processes: Potential trade-offs for the emotional and behavioral development of girls and boys. *Psychological Bulletin, 132*(1), 98–131. http://dx.doi.org/10.1037/0033-2909.132.1.98.

Rose, C. A., Simpson, C. G., & Moss, A. (2015). The bullying dynamic: Prevelance of involvement among a large-scale sample of middle and high school youth with and without disabilities. *Psychology in the Schools, 52*(5), 515–531. http://dx.doi.org/10.1002/pits.21840.

Rowley, E., Chandler, S., Baird, G., Simonoff, E., Pickles, A., Loucas, T., & Charman, T. (2012). The experience of friendship, victimization and bullying in children with an autism spectrum disorder: Associations with child characteristics and school placement. *Research in Autism Spectrum Disorders, 6*(3), 1126–1134. http://dx.doi.org/10.1016/j.rasd.2012.03.004.

Schwartz, D. (2000). Subtypes of victims and aggressors in children's peer groups. *Journal of Abnormal Child Psychology, 28*(2), 181–192. http://dx.doi.org/10.1023/A:1005174831561.

Schwartz, D., Farver, J. M., Chang, L., & Lee-Shin, Y. (2002). Victimization in South Korean children's peer groups. *Journal of Abnormal Child Psychology, 30*(2), 113–125. http://dx.doi.org/10.1023/a:1014749131245.

Schwartz, D., Proctor, L. J., & Chien, D. H. (2001). The aggressive victim of bullying: Emotional and behavioral dysregulation as a pathway to victimization by peers. In J. Juvonen, & S. Graham (Eds.), *Peer harassment in school: The plight of the vulnerable and victimized* (pp. 147–174). New York: Guilford.

Segers, M., & Rawana, J. (2014). What do we know about suicidality in autism spectrum disorders? A systematic review. *Autism Research, 7*(4), 507–521. http://dx.doi.org/10.1002/aur.1375.

Shattuck, P. T., Seltzer, M. M., Greenberg, J. S., Orsmond, G. I., Bolt, D., Kring, S., … Lord, C. (2007). Change in autism symptoms and maladaptive behaviors in adolescents and adults with an autism spectrum disorder. *Journal of Autism and Developmental Disorders, 37*(9), 1735–1747.

van Steensel, F. J., Bogels, S. M., & Perrin, S. (2011). Anxiety disorders in children and adolescents with autistic spectrum disorders: A meta-analysis. *Clinical Child and Family Psychology Review, 14*(3), 302–317. http://dx.doi.org/10.1007/s10567-011-0097-0.

Sterzing, P. R., Shattuck, P. T., Narendorf, S. C., Wagner, M., & Cooper, B. P. (2012). Bullying involvement and autism spectrum disorders. *Archives of Pediatrics and Adolescent Medicine, 166*(11), 1058–1064. http://dx.doi.org/10.1001/archpediatrics.2012.790.

Storch, E. A., Larson, M. J., Ehrenreich-May, J., Arnold, E. B., Jones, A. M., Renno, P., … Wood, J. J. (2012). Peer victimization in youth with autism spectrum disorders and co-occurring anxiety: Relations with psychopathology and loneliness. *Journal of Developmental and Physical Disabilities, 24*, 575–590.

Storch, E. A., Lewin, A. B., Collier, A. B., Arnold, E., De Nadai, A. S., … Murphy, T. K. (2015). A randomized controlled trial of cognitive-behavioral therapy versus treatment as usual for adolescents with autism spectrum disorders and comorbid anxiety. *Depression and Anxiety, 32*(3), 174–181. http://dx.doi.org/10.1002/da.22332.

Symes, W., & Humphrey, N. (2010). Peer-group indicators of social inclusion among pupils with autistic spectrum disorders (ASD) in mainstream secondary schools: A comparative study. *School Psychology International, 31*(5), 478–494. http://dx.doi.org/10.1177/0143034310382496.

Taylor, J. L., & Gotham, K. O. (2016). Cumulative life events, traumatic experiences, and psychiatric symptomatology in transition-aged youth with autism spectrum disorder. *Journal of Neurodevelopmental Disorders, 8*(1), 28. http://dx.doi.org/10.1186/s11689-016-9160-y.

Taylor, J. L., & Mailick, M. R. (2014). A longitudinal examination of 10-year change in vocational and educational activities for adults with autism spectrum disorders. *Developmental Psychology, 50*(3), 699–708. http://dx.doi.org/10.1037/a0034297.

Taylor, J. L., McPheeters, M. L., Sathe, N. A., Dove, D., Veenstra-Vanderweele, J., & Warren, Z. (2012). A systematic review of vocational interventions for young adults with autism spectrum disorders. *Pediatrics, 130*(3), 531–538. http://dx.doi.org/10.1542/peds.2012-0682.

Twyman, K. A., Saylor, C. F., Saia, D., Macias, M. M., Taylor, L. A., & Spratt, E. (2010). Bullying and ostracism experiences in children with special health care needs. *Journal of Developmental and Behavioral Pediatrics, 31*(1), 1–8. http://dx.doi.org/10.1097/DBP.0b013e3181c828c8.

Wainscot, J. J., Naylor, P., Sutcliffe, P., Tantam, D., & Williams, J. V. (2008). Relationships with peers and use of the school environment of mainstream secondary school pupils with Asperger syndrome (high-functioning autism): A case-control study. *International Journal of Psychology & Psychological Therapy, 8*(1), 25–38.

Whitehouse, A. J. O., Durkin, K., Jaquet, E., & Ziatas, K. (2009). Friendship, loneliness and depression in adolescents with Asperger's syndrome. *Journal of Adolescence, 32*(2), 309–322. http://dx.doi.org/10.1016/j.adolescence.2008.03.004.

Williams, K. D. (2007). Ostracism. *Annual Review of Psychology, 58*(1), 425–452. http://dx.doi.org/10.1146/annurev.psych.58.110405.085641.

Wood, J. J., Ehrenreich-May, J., Alessandri, M., Fujii, C., Renno, P., Laugeson, E., … Storch, E. A. (2015). Cognitive behavioral therapy for early adolescents with autism spectrum disorders and clinical anxiety: A randomized, controlled trial. *Behavior Therapy, 46*(1), 7–19. http://dx.doi.org/10.1016/j.beth.2014.01.002.

Yeager, D. S., Fong, C. J., Lee, H. Y., & Espelage, D. L. (2015). Declines in efficacy of anti-bullying programs among older adolescents: Theory and a three-level meta-analysis. *Journal of Applied Developmental Psychology, 37*, 36–51. http://dx.doi.org/10.1037/a0023626.10.1037/0022-0167.26.5.4591979-34224-001.

Zeedyk, S. M., Rodriguez, G., Tipton, L. A., Baker, B. L., & Blacher, J. (2014). Bullying of youth with autism spectrum disorder, intellectual disability, or typical development: Victim and parent perspectives. *Research in Autism Spectrum Disorders, 8*(9), 1173–1183. http://dx.doi.org/10.1016/j.rasd.2014.06.001.

CHAPTER FOUR

Video-Based Group Instruction for Adolescents With Autism Spectrum Disorders: A Case of Intervention Development

Joshua B. Plavnick[1], **Brooke Ingersoll**
Michigan State University, East Lansing, MI, United States
[1]Corresponding author: E-mail: plavnick@msu.edu

Contents

Abstract

Social interaction skills are critical indicators of positive life outcomes across multiple domains of functioning for adolescents diagnosed with an autism spectrum disorder (ASD). To date, intervention research has provided very few community-based social skills treatment options for service providers of adolescents with ASD. This chapter documents a case example of intervention development designed to address the

International Review of Research in Developmental Disabilities, Volume 52
ISSN 2211-6095
http://dx.doi.org/10.1016/bs.irrdd.2017.07.002

gap in empirically supported social skills training programs for the aforementioned subgroup of adolescents with ASD while following recent guidelines from implementation science (Fixsen, Naoom, Blasé, Friedman, & Wallace, 2005) and contextually based ASD intervention development (Dingfelder & Mandell, 2011; Kasari & Smith, 2013). We describe an iterative process of contextually driven development of a social skills instruction program for adolescents with ASD in a public high school, which can serve as a model for the development of sustainable intervention.

Social impairments are a hallmark feature of autism spectrum disorders (ASDs), and some suggest that they are the defining feature of the disorder (Gillis, Callahan, & Romanczyk, 2011). As children age, social skills are closely tied to quality of life and affect levels of community inclusion (Orsmond, Krauss, & Seltzer, 2004), occupational functioning (Rao, Beidel, & Murray, 2008), and independent living (Howlin, Goode, Hutton, & Rutter, 2004) among individuals with ASD. In addition, studies examining the course of ASD symptoms over the life span suggest that most individuals with ASD continue to show significant social difficulties in adolescence and adulthood (Seltzer, Shattuck, Abbeduto, & Greenberg, 2004).

Advocacy groups, such as Autism Speaks, and funding agencies, such as the National Institutes of Health and Institute of Education Science, have recently supported increased research attention to develop effective interventions for older individuals with ASD, with social interaction being a primary objective in many calls for research (Odom, Duda, Kucharczyk, Cox, & Stable, 2014). However, the mere development of interventions, without considering current and future contexts for intervention and implementers, is not likely to create desired changes and lead to long-term adoption, utilization, and sustainability (Dingfelder & Mandell, 2011). We believe there is value for intervention developers who see early tests of efficacy through to sustained implementation within the location where those tests occur. Traditionally, developers test their interventions in service delivery settings and then may or may not support communities in sustaining those interventions following preliminary research efforts (Kasari & Smith, 2013). Failing to collect the important information that can only be derived from ongoing implementation may limit the extent to which the intervention is developed in a manner that will support its long-term use.

The objective of this chapter is to discuss a case example of the development of a social skills intervention for adolescents with ASD that was directly informed by an implementation science framework originally outlined by Fixsen et al. (2005) and recommendations for ASD intervention development by Dingfelder and Mandell (2011) and Kasari and Smith (2013). The implementation science perspective emphasizes the need to use evidence-based implementation practices to embed an established practice within an existing entity (e.g., a public school). Without evidence-based implementation practices, evidence-based practices cannot traverse the research to practice gap. Although not specific to implementation of interventions for children with ASD, the stages of implementation and core implementation components align with several recent recommendations for effective ASD intervention design and early implementation (Cook & Odom, 2013; Dingfelder & Mandell, 2011; Kasari & Smith, 2013). The implementation science perspective combined with the recent recommendations for ASD intervention developers may collectively inform methods researchers can take during the early development process to develop a usable and acceptable intervention (Dingfelder and Mandell) that is designed for implementation and scaling (Fixsen et al., 2005).

The intervention in the present case example, video-based group instruction (VGI), was developed in collaboration with public school professionals to meet the contextual demands associated with high school settings, where the majority of adolescents with ASD receive services and opportunities to interact socially with peers. The goal of the collaboration was to create an intervention that would then be sustained by educational personnel and potentially transferred to other educational environments. The present paper contributes to recent ASD intervention development literature by explicitly describing the ongoing development process in relation to a specific intervention. First, we provide background information on the research to practice gap for many empirically validated ASD interventions. We then describe implementation stages and the core components necessary for effective implementation (Fixsen et al., 2005) and outline how these components informed our process of early development and implementation of VGI. Finally, we discuss how our experiences with research and development of a school-based social skills intervention may inform other intervention developers.

1. INTERVENTION RESEARCH TO PRACTICE GAPS

Within the context of evidence-based practice for youth with ASD, researchers have categorized practices into focused and comprehensive interventions (Odom, Boyd, Hall, & Hume, 2010). Focused interventions typically target a specific behavior, are administered for a small duration of the day, and occur over a brief period of time (Odom et al.). Examples include video modeling, peer-mediated intervention, and reinforcement. Comprehensive interventions are defined as a combined set of manualized procedures with the intent of having a broad impact on several behavioral and psychosocial outcomes (Odom et al.). Comprehensive interventions are often administered for at least one year and with intensity greater than 20 h per week. Examples include the Early Start Denver Model, the UCLA Young Autism Project, and the Princeton Child Development Institute. Some interventions may have characteristics of both focused and comprehensive interventions as focused interventions can combine multiple procedures and be administered over an extended period of time (e.g., 1 year), though they do not meet the intensity requirement of a comprehensive intervention.

Focused interventions are often investigated using single-case experimental designs, with multiple high-quality replications of a particular practice or intervention package leading to eventual nomination as an evidence-based practice (Odom et al., 2010). Selection of such practices is recommended over other practices with less evidence in most situations, though a provider's knowledge of the child and environment also play an important role in the delivery of procedures (Slocum et al., 2014). One difficulty practitioners face in translating evidence-based practices into day-to-day implementation is that the practitioner's environment (e.g., public school) may or may not align with the environments in which the intervention was previously tested (Wood, McLeod, Klebanoff, & Brookman-Frazee, 2015). In addition, interventionists often need to combine or dismantle components of interventions reported in the literature, and the extent to which adaptations will lead to positive outcomes for the recipient have rarely been empirically tested.

A second dilemma is somewhat more nuanced and involves the process by which single-case research is carried out. Most single-case studies are administered for a relatively brief portion of the day (e.g., 30 min is a long session) and over a short duration, such as 3–6 months. However, educators may need procedures that fit into different time frames, such as a 1-h high school period, and want to administer an intervention for the entire year. Although individuals with a vast understanding of the broader literature may be able to recombine interventions examined in various studies, community service providers may not have the training or time to do so. As such, it may be difficult for community providers to implement focused interventions with fidelity to the procedures reported in published literature. And yet, it is often not known whether modified interventions incorporate the essential features of a published study. These factors can be barriers to practitioners' successful implementation of evidence-based focused interventions for individuals with ASD.

Historically, comprehensive interventions for individuals with ASD have been designed and initially implemented in research settings, following the "stage pipeline"—a series of efficacy studies in clinical or research settings, culminating in a final effectiveness study in the community (Rohrbach, Grana, Sussman, & Valente, 2006; T. Smith et al., 2007). As described by T. Smith et al. (2007), the process begins with highly controlled studies that demonstrate an intervention leads to positive outcomes (i.e., efficacy). Researchers then gradually transfer control of implementing the intervention to service providers in the targeted service delivery settings and assess outcomes (i.e., effectiveness). When the "stage pipeline" progression was originally proposed, there were very few rigorous between-group studies examining interventions for individuals with ASD, and an emphasis was placed on addressing such a limitation. However, in the years that followed, several randomized controlled trials of ASD interventions were conducted and a new problem emerged; once implemented in the community, interventions were often not as effective and frequently did not sustain over time (e.g., Suhrheinrich et al., 2013). Thus, there has been a call for intervention developers in the field to incorporate features into the initial intervention and study design that will cultivate its ongoing use and effectiveness in broad contexts (Dingfelder & Mandell, 2011).

Across comprehensive and focused interventions, recent recommendations in the field move researchers away from a tightly controlled progression of development and study toward an approach that considers the terminal implementation setting from the earliest stages of development (Dingfelder & Mandell, 2011; Kasari & Smith, 2013). Although carefully controlled studies may allow researchers to definitively test an intervention, the absence of relevant contextual variables often produce limited effectiveness data. Dingfelder and Mandell propose applying the diffusion of innovation theory (Rogers, 2003) to the autism field, which includes involving local stakeholders in all steps of the research and development process, as well as a process to make successive modifications to the intervention as problems of fit are identified across studies and communities. For example, prior to and during a study of a social skills intervention implemented in a school setting by school personnel, researchers would involve families, teachers, clinicians, and administrators in the development of the research agenda. The process or "pipeline" is adjusted to ensure that there is a link between intervention development and the settings in which the interventions are most likely to be used.

These concepts are echoed by Kasari and Smith (2013), who also recommend testing interventions in the context in which they will be used from the initial stages. Kasari and Smith propose starting with a "partial effectiveness" trial where researchers carry out the intervention in the school setting. This allows the intervention to be tested in context, thus providing a demonstration of efficacy in the school setting before community providers are expected to implement. Dingfelder and Mandell (2011) and Kasari and Smith (2013) both speak to the need for development of interventions within the contexts where they will be implemented. Otherwise, highly efficacious interventions will continue to be reported in research literature, though these interventions may not be adopted in community settings or, when adopted, the effectiveness of the interventions may suffer.

Both focused and comprehensive interventions suffer from issues pertaining to contextual fit and implementation. In some cases, interventions have been developed in idiosyncratic environments and for various reasons (e.g., staffing ratios, administrative support) fail to transfer when deployed in community settings. In such cases, the issue is one of development and requires intervention developers include considerations of community environments during the development process (Dingfelder & Mandell, 2011; Kasari & Smith, 2013). In other cases, interventions have been developed with community input yet suffer from issues pertaining to implementation, which limits the extent to which the practice will be sustained or scaled (Odom et al., 2014). Each of these issues has been extensively investigated by implementation scientists across a number of human service domains.

2. IMPLEMENTATION SCIENCE AND INTERVENTION DEVELOPMENT

Fixsen et al. (2005) outlined stages of implementation and core implementation components that offer specific and systematic approaches to the widespread implementation of practices. The implementation stages, outlined in Table 1, describe a temporal sequence of events beginning with exploration and ending with sustainability. Based on their review of

Table 1 Stages of Implementation Defined

Stage	Definition
Exploration and adoption	Assess potential match between community needs, community resources, and an evidence-based program. Understand the enabling and limiting needs of a community for a specific intervention.
Program installation	Structural supports, such as funding, human resources, policy changes, and reporting guidelines, necessary to support a program are put in place.
Initial implementation	The changes in daily behaviors of purveyors that align with carrying out a new practice. This stage often involves ongoing education and training.
Full operation	All staff members are hired and trained and begin implementing the intervention as daily practice. All relevant clients or students receive the intervention. It typically takes 2–4 years to reach this stage.
Innovation	Changes in the practice occurring at a specific site, including both undesired drift and desired innovations.
Sustainability	Ongoing use of the intervention as staff and administrators leave positions and are replaced by new personnel, and as policy changes occur inside and outside of the organization.

the research literature, the timeline for an agency to start and progress through the implementation process is approximately 2–4 years.

The core implementation components compliment the stages by outlining the necessary elements for a successful implementation (Fixsen et al., 2005). Components include the following:

1. Selection or hiring of staff who are qualified to carry out the intervention.
2. Preservice training that ensures staff learn the reasons why a practice is important and learn to implement procedures with fidelity.
3. Ongoing coaching to ensure staff change previous behaviors and sustain accurate implementation.
4. Staff evaluation to determine whether the hiring and training processes worked as intended.
5. Program evaluation to assess whether the organization changes its behavior to ensure accurate sustained implementation.

6. Facilitative administration to review data produced by the program and make data-based decisions to best support sustained implementation of a practice.
7. Systems interventions to ensure external systems (e.g., financial, policy) continue to support implementation.

Most intervention development research involves some aspects of the first four implementation components, with little inclusion of the final three components. But we offer that it can be beneficial for intervention developers to understand how each component works on a small scale (e.g., within a single service location) for a particular intervention being developed. Doing so may alter the final version of the intervention in a manner that is more useful to final consumers.

Over the past 5 years, we have been working on the development of a social skills intervention designed for implementation in a public high school setting for adolescents with ASD. VGI is a multicomponent social skills group that utilizes concepts, principles, and procedures from applied behavior analysis including video modeling, direct instruction, differential reinforcement, token economies, performance feedback, multiple exemplar training, and natural environment training to promote social functioning (Plavnick, Sam, Hume, & Odom, 2013). VGI can be considered a focused intervention, though it is designed for delivery over an entire school year, with social targets added over time, similar to other curricular targets in educational settings. As a result, the need to consider evidence-based implementation practices as the intervention was installed in a school setting was essential to meet the demands of our consumers.

Broadly speaking, VGI is a social skills group designed for a small homogeneous sample of adolescents with ASD and consisting of three main components: (1) direct instruction to label, define, and follow basic social rules (e.g., looking at people when talking to them); (2) targeted video modeling to teach complex social interactions with peers (e.g., multicomponent initiations directed toward multiple peers involved in an activity); and (3) natural environment training to practice social rules and complex social behaviors. The development process combines recommendations from T. Smith et al. (2007) as well as more recent recommendations for contextually driven development (e.g., Dingfelder & Mandell, 2011). In addition, because the goal has been to create a contextually relevant and efficacious procedure likely to be sustained in schools, our development process adopted an implementation science framework (Fixsen et al., 2005).

3. COMMUNITY-BASED VIDEO-BASED GROUP INSTRUCTION RESEARCH AND DEVELOPMENT

Intervention development raises several important questions including (1) identifying components that make up the intervention package, (2) determining whether the intervention is socially valid to consumers, (3) determining whether the package works and which components are essential, (4) determining if it is feasible for providers to implement, and (5) identifying the best methods to train providers to implement the intervention (Dingfelder & Mandell, 2011). We believe that the starting point in the process outlined above may vary from one development project to the next, likely due to differences in the extent to which the intervention or its components are already developed and the identified implementation site (e.g., schools, independent living homes, community service agencies). Further, intervention developers are likely to find that answering one question may have implications for the procedures involved in answering another; for example, identification of essential components must be informed by social validity. However, social validity may vary based on a particular consumer group and could potentially change after effective training methods are developed and administered. As a result, intervention developers likely need to evaluate the context within which their intervention will be delivered and identify the most appropriate path of development that leads to a feasible, efficacious, and socially valid intervention.

Ultimately, intervention developers must walk a careful line to ensure their proposed procedures can be efficacious and simultaneously ensure consumers will adopt and implement those procedures in the service setting. Should researchers plan to follow such a progression toward demonstrating community effectiveness, as illustrated in this article, there are a number of factors to consider. Though certainly not exhaustive, several of the considerations that were key throughout this development process are described below and outlined in Table 2 along with the corresponding areas of concern and suggestions proposed by Dingfelder and Mandell, 2011.

3.1 Early Development

Developing an intervention that is likely to be adopted requires that even early stages of efficacy research be conducted in natural settings with community partners (Kasari & Smith, 2013). As described previously, the current status of intervention research in ASD, including studies involving social skills instruction, indicates that once an intervention is operationalized and

Table 2 Alignment Between Intervention Development Recommendations and Video-Based Group Instruction (VGI) Development Procedures

Intervention Development Suggestions (Dingfelder & Mandell, 2011)	VGI Development Procedures
Involve community members in the research from the beginning	Intervention testing took place in a school setting, administered by a local service provider; researchers met with teacher and paraprofessionals prior to intervention implementation to seek feedback on protocol elements
Build on existing community relationships	Implementation of VGI in public school district where investigators had previous research relationship
Conduct a community analysis to identify key opinion leaders and other potential community partners	Principal investigator met with district administration to discuss range of options before settling on developing a VGI class within the high school setting
Use change agents as "boundary spanners" to develop community relationships	Teachers with previous relationships with research staff helped coordinate implementation in school setting
Develop intervention for behaviors most salient to the public	Social impairment is a hallmark feature of ASD; individuals with ASD continue to show social difficulties throughout their lives
Elicit guidance from administrators and families to encourage faithfulness to the principles guiding the treatment protocol	Principal investigator met with district and school administration, as well as the facilitator, to ensure daily implementation of the complete package could occur
Ensure goodness of fit with clinical setting, interventionists, and clients	VGI was designed for group administration to fit within the constraints of a typical high school classroom; parents contributed to dependent variable selection
Continually modify intervention as problems are identified by interventionists	Protocol was shortened to a 50-min session to fit within the average class period; alterations to initial procedures were made to increase feasibility of implementation for teacher in school setting (see Table 3)
Continue to work with administrators, practitioners, and families to assess long-term feasibility of the protocol	Principal investigator obtained ongoing feedback from many consumers (e.g., parents, participants, teachers, administrators) to continuously assess sustained implementation

Identify long-term demands of treatment	A preliminary feasibility study assessed levels of external support necessary to ensure sustained implementation with fidelity
Build data collection mechanisms into intervention protocol	Data on client outcomes was collected live by the group leader, precluding the necessity of video cameras or observation windows; implementation checklists were built into the training and coaching protocols
Recruit a sample representative of all children with ASD	Research studies to date have targeted a specific subgroup of individuals with ASD, a diverse sample of this subgroup has been recruited across studies
Report exclusions, participation rates, dropouts, and representativeness on key characteristics	Specific inclusion criteria has been developed and reported in research studies published to date
Measure outcomes relevant to the intervention setting	Parents and facilitator suggested various target behaviors for future emphasis, which were then added to the protocol
Assess treatment adoption	Feasibility of implementation was assessed using procedural integrity checklists; teachers were interviewed following implementation to assess likelihood of sustained use
Describe characteristics of practitioners and compare to interventionists who will eventually implement the intervention in the community	Characteristics of practitioners have been described; teacher implementation fits with predicted community implementers
Include interventionists with a variety of background/experience, and report on differences related to said background	First interventionist had training in applied behavior analysis, whereas second interventionist did not
Collect data on likely treatment demands, such as time, staffing, parent involvement required, and total cost of implementation	Staffing demands and time for preparation and implementation were assessed using time logs and teacher interviews
Implement community-based effectiveness trials	VGI was tested with one local high school teacher to determine effectiveness of implementation before planned expansion

ASD, autism spectrum disorder.

leaves the confines of the developer's clinic or model program, implementation with fidelity in naturalistic settings may be difficult (Odom et al., 2014). It is, however, implementation in those naturalistic settings that is required to support skill maintenance, generalization, and overall effects (Gresham, Sugai, & Horner, 2001). Most service delivery settings are complicated environments, pushed by the demands of everyday life. Interventions and experimental methodologies created for a controlled setting are ill-equipped for the challenges of most service delivery settings (Berliner, 2002).

During both efficacy and effectiveness studies, as well as during replication and broader dissemination, intervention developers may benefit by considering the skills and resources of staff, potential barriers to implementation, and the fit between the community partners and the intervention (Fixsen et al., 2005). In the case of a public school, this can be achieved through systematically involving caregivers, practitioners, students, and administrators throughout the intervention and study design process using activities such as interviews and focus groups to provide opportunities for feedback on materials and tools; creating alliances across these multiple stakeholders; building an implementation team that includes stakeholders; and gathering frequent social validity data to assess the fit of the intervention with community priorities, needs, and available resources. In addition, selecting intervention outcomes that match the needs of stakeholders is critical to supporting initial adoption of interventions and maintenance over time (Dingfelder & Mandell, 2011).

3.1.1 Preliminary Investigation of Video-Based Group Instruction

Early development of VGI involved a partnership with community members, highlighted by preintervention interviews with parents of adolescents with ASD to assess critical social behaviors for the targeted subgroup and ongoing debrief sessions with the teacher who would facilitate the first iteration to understand barriers to successful implementation. These partnerships were based on recommendations of Dingfelder and Mandell (2011) to understand the resources available to community partners (e.g., organizational capacity, financing, policies) as well as the values and beliefs of key community partners including caregivers and service providers (Dingfelder & Mandell, 2011). The inclusion of community partners allowed the researchers to quickly and adeptly make modifications to the intervention that would ease transport into future community settings. For example, the facilitator and parents all suggested emphasizing target behaviors pertaining to initiations of conventional social interaction, such as commenting or showing others items of interest. Although not originally targeted as part of VGI, each of these behaviors was added to the initial teaching list of target behaviors for future iterations. This addition was supported by post-intervention social validity data, in which all responding teachers and parents rated the targeted behaviors as being very important to the participants.

In addition to guidance from Dingfelder and Mandell (2011), the suggestion of T. Smith et al. (2007) to conduct initial efficacy studies of the intervention or components of the intervention was also incorporated in the early development process of VGI. A single-case experimental design was used to conduct an initial efficacy study of using video modeling to teach the targeted social skills to groups of adolescents with ASD. Although video modeling had prior evidence of efficacy (Bellini, Peters, Benner, & Hopf, 2007), it had been minimally applied to small groups of learners, which was a necessity for feasible implementation within public school settings. During the initial test of VGI, the procedure was implemented 2 days a week in a school setting, though after school hours. One reason for this approach was to ensure participants acquired the targeted behaviors using the planned instructional procedures before approaching school personnel about using educational time to administer the intervention. A second reason was to test the feasibility of delivery by an educator who received training in the protocol but was not a highly trained doctoral research assistant or behavior analyst, thereby planning ahead for intervention maintenance and sustainability. Collectively, the early development process allowed for intervention development informed by consumers, initial efficacy of the core component (video modeling) when used for small group instruction, and a partial assessment of feasibility of implementation.

In sum, the community-based collaborations during the early stages of development helped create a bridge from the initial assessment (i.e., Plavnick et al., 2013) to implementation in a public school setting as intended (discussed below). Employing and training a teacher as the facilitator in the initial study, prepared researchers for future training needs. In addition, obtaining feedback from parents of participants provided critical information about the goals, procedures, and outcomes of VGI. This information was combined with data derived from formal and informal meetings with educators to establish guidelines for initial implementation in the schools. These guidelines were built into procedural revisions, implementation checklists, and the training and coaching protocols that would be used across subsequent stages of development.

3.1.2 Adapting Video-Based Group Instruction for Implementation Within the School Setting

As discussed by Dingfelder and Mandell (2011), the critical components of adoption involve relative advantage of an intervention over the current practice, the compatibility of the procedures with the culture of the intervention setting, and the complexity of the intervention in terms of a usability perspective. As such, we decided the second critical step in the development of VGI was to deliver the intervention within the public high school context. The process of identifying a partnering school was careful and systematic, with the goal of finding a district where the procedures could eventually be supported independent of the investigators.

Selection of the school and preliminary relationship development were critical preparation components that went into the second iteration (see exploration stage of implementation in Fixsen et al., 2005). The first author developed a research relationship with a local public school district and met with district level administrators to discuss the possibility of implementing VGI at one of the local high schools. Once administrative support was established, the first author met multiple times with the teachers who would implement the procedures with students to discuss specific logistics pertaining to carrying out implementation sessions within classrooms. Kasari and Smith (2013) recommend involving teachers from early stages in the development and study of intervention as a way to avoid "...becoming committed to an intervention that is not well matched to ...teachers in the school" (p. 26). The teachers were instrumental in the revision process as they were best suited to identify components that had to be altered for sustained implementation. In essence, it was the teachers who would make decisions about whether VGI demonstrated relative advantage over current practices was compatible with the culture of existing programs and was not too complex to be usable (critical components introduced by Dingfelder & Mandell, 2011). An informal meeting was conducted wherein researchers introduced the intervention to educators (i.e., teachers and paraprofessionals in the classrooms) and sought feedback on elements that required modification.

There is an ongoing discussion in the literature about fidelity and adaptation (Blakely et al., 1987; Smith, Daunic, and Taylor, 2007), or "finding the right mix of fidelity and adaptation" (Durlak & DuPre, 2008). Researchers must try to balance the need for determining efficacy while considering appropriate adaptations for specific communities. Teams may consider the following strategies to balance the fidelity/adaption debate: (1) if researchers are knowledgeable about their communities, as proposed above, they should be able to modify a program to make it more effective in a specific context and (2) intervention developers should identify the theoretically essential or core components of the intervention that most directly link to outcomes. The meetings with educators prior to implementation of VGI in the school setting allowed for an informed adaptation process that blended the core components identified by the researchers with the cultural and practical needs of the school.

The most important adaptation as VGI was moved into a public school site was to fit procedures within a typical school schedule. VGI was therefore adjusted from a 75-min to 50-min session, but now delivered every day as opposed to 2 days each week. Functionally speaking, it became a class for the students who participated in the session. The changes in timing of group administration would prove to be an important adjustment to the long-term implementation of the program within the school, though brought several logistical challenges that needed to be addressed and studied.

Although the overall weekly time for sessions increased, the decrease in session length meant fewer learning opportunities within that session for each participant to practice the targeted skills. High rates of learning opportunities are very important for individuals with more severe disabilities, particularly as they learn new skills (Weinkauf, Zeug, Anderson, & Ala'i-Rosales, 2011). It was unknown whether the reduction in session-by-session learning opportunities would interfere with participants learning new social skills. To ensure that learning continued at an acceptable rate despite lowering the number of learning opportunities for each participant within a session, we planned to continuously monitor the number of trials before participants reached a predetermined performance criterion. Individualized adaptations could then be made for participants who did not demonstrate progress toward that criterion at a rate similar to participants in the previous investigation.

The second critical adaptation was to reduce the complexity of the intervention without compromising the essential features. The teacher implementing VGI had less experience with applied behavior analysis than the facilitator in the first iteration. Many components of the intervention including the token economy, direct instruction, video modeling, differential reinforcement, error correction, prompt fading, and systematic data-based decision-making were relatively novel tasks for the new facilitator, as they likely would be for many educators. Careful adaptations were therefore made to "meet the communities' needs and capabilities"

(Dingfelder & Mandell, 2011, p. 607). To reduce complexity, each component of VGI was assessed and simplified whenever possible. For example, instead of creating a token economy system associated with following the rules of social skills group from the outset, educators were trained to provide preferred snacks when students demonstrated behavior that aligned with selected rules. The token economy required conditioning stimuli, such as points, as reinforcers. The added step of conditioning a reinforcer increased complexity and was therefore added later in the implementation process, as the teacher demonstrated high levels of proficiency and indicated she was comfortable with the other components of the group. Table 3 outlines adaptations made to simplify VGI without compromising the core components for the second iteration.

3.2 Implementing and Evaluating Iterations of the Intervention

As development of VGI progressed from the initial study through collaborative planning with educators in a public school implementation site, two semester-long studies were conducted to further develop the intervention procedures. During the first semester, we evaluated the level of support educators required to implement the revised components with fidelity. We also examined the feasibility of administering VGI to adolescents with more severe ASD. A second study was then conducted to evaluate the efficacy of the now-abbreviated intervention for adolescent participants when a public school teacher implemented procedures with high integrity.

3.2.1 Study 1: Training, Coaching, and Fidelity of Implementation

The facilitators for the second iteration were two trained special educators with experience teaching secondary students with ASD. Adolescent participants between 14 and 18 years of age were referred by each teacher. Participants were divided into homogenous groups by researchers and teachers based on severity of intellectual disability. As a result, one group contained one female and three male participants with mild to moderate intellectual disability and ASD, while the second group contained two female and two male participants with moderate to severe intellectual disability and ASD. The latter group also demonstrated more severe social deficits. Target behaviors were selected for each group based on common social deficits identified across group members by both teachers and researchers prior to intervention.

Table 3 Description and Rationale for Modifications Made After Initial Implementation

Element	Initial Implementation	Adjustment	Reason for Change
Setting	Administered in a classroom after school hours with no other students present.	Administered in a classroom during the school day with students in and out of room.	Initial assessment of procedures with reduced distractions and immediate follow-up in setting more similar to typical implementation.
Assessments	The ASSP was administered prior to the start of VGI. A satisfaction survey was administered to parents at end of VGI.	ADOS, WASI, and ASSP were administered prior to the start of VGI.	Ensure participants met inclusion criteria of ASD/ID
Session length	75-min sessions 2 days a week	50-min sessions delivered every day	Altered to fit into school environment (i.e., sessions delivered as "class")
Learning opportunities	Rapid pace of instruction during review of rules and 10 trials for targeted behaviors during video modeling	Slower pace of instruction during review of rules and 6–8 trials for targeted behaviors during video modeling	Interventionist required practice to administer rule review learning opportunities at rapid pace. Video modeling trials reduced due reduction in session length.
Data collection	Facilitator collected data on whether participants watched the video.	Facilitator did not collect data on whether participants watched the video.	Ease implementation for facilitator during early stages of training.

(*Continued*)

Table 3 Description and Rationale for Modifications Made After Initial Implementation—cont'd

Element	Initial Implementation	Adjustment	Reason for Change
Token economy	Participants earned points for following rules throughout the sessions and had an opportunity to trade in points.	For the first half of VGI, participants earned edibles for following rules. A token economy was introduced halfway through VGI and tokens were traded in for preferred items.	Stagger introduction of components to ease implementation of novel tasks for facilitator.
Rule review	Facilitator collected data on whether participants followed the rules and had criteria for selecting new rules.	Facilitator did not collect data during rule review and rules modified as suggested by researchers.	Ease implementation for facilitator by reducing overall amount of data and adjustments to procedures.

ASD, autism spectrum disorder; *ASSP*, autism social skills profile; *ID*, intellectual disability; *VGI*, video-based group instruction.

Preparation of educators to implement the program required initial didactic instruction with role-play, followed by ongoing coaching to ensure accurate implementation and data collection. Ongoing coaching followed guidelines set forth by Fixsen, Blase, Naoom, and Wallace (2009) and started with alternated instruction, wherein the program developer and teacher alternated back and forth during an instructional session. This format provided a model of the procedure and an opportunity for the teacher to implement the procedure with immediate feedback from the developer. The alternations gave way to independent implementation with the researcher providing vocal coaching and end-of-session feedback. Vocal coaching was gradually faded over a two-week period as the teacher demonstrated accurate implementation. At this time, the program developer or a research assistant observed two sessions each week and provided postsession feedback from data collected via a 41-item procedural integrity checklist (available from first author). Implementation outcomes were reviewed with the teacher immediately following an observation period. Procedural integrity outcomes were observed to gradually increase from 71% at the beginning of a semester to 86% at the end of the semester, with a mean of 81% accurate implementation across the entire semester.

Both educators were able to administer VGI sessions with fidelity. However, only one group of participants demonstrated gains in the social behaviors that were targeted within VGI sessions. None of the participants in the group with moderate to severe intellectual disability demonstrated increased levels of social skills as a result of VGI. Although we did not empirically evaluate the reasons why this group was not successful, we hypothesize that some adolescents will continue to require very low student to teacher ratios (e.g., one to one) and extensive learning opportunities to demonstrate acquisition of novel social interaction skills. Conversely, the group with mild to moderate intellectual disability demonstrated gains in social interaction skills targeted during the social skills group. Over a 12-week period, the three participants met acquisition criteria (i.e., 80% correct responding over two consecutive sessions) for eight targeted social skills. The results suggested teachers could implement procedures with fidelity to the developed intervention and that individuals who had demonstrated success learning within a group context may be optimal participants for the VGI program as developed.

3.2.2 Study 2: School-Based Experimental Analysis

Teachers demonstrated they could reliably implement VGI in Study 1. In addition, participants with ASD and mild to moderate intellectual disability acquired targeted behaviors, while participants with more severe intellectual disability did not. Therefore, we conducted a second study to experimentally evaluate the effects of VGI on adolescents with ASD and mild to moderate intellectual disability when implemented by a teacher in a public school setting.

Four adolescents (two males and two females) with ASD and mild to moderate intellectual disability who had not participated in the initial implementation phase were recruited for the efficacy study (see Plavnick, Kaid, & MacFarland, 2015). One of the teachers from the preceding study facilitated VGI with the new group of adolescent participants. Similar to the previous phase, VGI was administered on a daily basis for 50-min sessions. Additionally, the same behaviors administered to the group with moderate intellectual disability in the preceding study were targeted for this investigation, which reduced the amount of coaching the teacher needed to administer VGI. A single-case multiple probe across behaviors design was used to experimentally evaluate the effects of VGI on the acquisition of targeted behaviors. For the most part, outcomes replicated the original investigation (Plavnick et al., 2013) and speak of the potential of VGI as a social skills training program for a subgroup of adolescents with ASD in public school settings. Additionally, social validity data showed robust agreement on the importance of the targeted behaviors as well as perception of the participants' enjoyment. All participating teachers and parents reported that they would recommend the program to others.

At the conclusion of the second semester, we had taught two educators to implement VGI to 11 adolescents with ASD, with seven adolescents demonstrating acquisition of targeted skills. We had identified several important refinements for future iterations. A common next step in the development of ASD interventions would be to recruit additional sites for participation to expand the scope of the intervention and assess whether a larger sample of participants were successful when the intervention was administered. Although this would be a long-term goal of VGI, we also had questions about the sustained implementation of this intervention within the school environment in which it had been placed. We believed the data that emerged from investigating an intervention within a site over time could lead to important intervention refinements that would improve its efficacy and effectiveness when taken to scale. We therefore conducted multiple interviews with educators and district administrators to obtain feedback on the procedure and outcomes and to understand what was necessary for the school to continue the intervention.

3.2.3 Consumer Feedback

Feedback from relevant stakeholders is an essential component of sustained implementation and, to the extent that the feedback is generalizable to other similar stakeholders, can support the development of more broadly usable interventions (Fixsen et al., 2005). During our interviews with educators who had been involved in implementing VGI, we learned that they liked the structure of the intervention and that the procedures called for daily implementation. The teachers indicated that they were interested in continuing the intervention, believed it was beneficial for participants, and asked if they would have support from researchers to continue implementation in the following academic year. In addition, teachers noted several areas that were important for us to learn and consider as we refined the intervention. First, teachers asked for additional video modeling content that they could use in a variety of settings and scenarios. Second, teachers indicated the need for participants to learn skills that would lead to their success when interacting with other adolescents in the school, across a variety of settings. Finally, teachers indicated the importance of increasing the group size to five or six adolescents and to expand participants beyond individuals with ASD to those with intellectual disability to include additional facilitators who served students with ASD within the school.

During interviews with district administrators, we learned that the school district had goals for special education programming at the high school level that could align with daily implementation of VGI and with the teacher-requested modifications. Administrators were specifically interested in the development of a peer-mediated intervention program at the high school level. The administration indicated a willingness to create an elective course for eligible students who took the peer-mediated intervention course. Doing so would create a mechanism to administer the VGI program to adolescents with disabilities with their typically developing peers in a manner that would be sustainable within the broader school framework.

Several planned changes emerged from the information gathered from school personnel. Decisions to make changes based on this feedback were consistent with the innovation stage of implementation (Fixsen et al., 2005) and incorporated Dingfelder and Mandell's (2011) suggestion to change interventions based on interventionist feedback. First, we decided to expand group sizes to six participants. Second, we created a series of additional videos that could be available to educators. Third, we added typically developing peers to a portion of the VGI session so that adolescents with disabilities could practice their acquired skills with typical peers. Each of these refinements was tested with pilot investigations to ensure outcomes were similar to previous investigations.

3.2.4 Study 3: Expanding Participation

As in previous iterations, a single-case experiment was planned to test the increased group sizes with participants of various disabilities. The study examined the application of VGI across two social skills groups, each consisting of six adolescents with varied intellectual and developmental disabilities. Researchers worked with teachers who had administered VGI in the preceding year to train and prepare two new educators to administer the intervention sessions.

Social skills groups operated in the same manner as the school-based groups described previously. Social skill acquisition was the primary variable of interest, with careful attention to the rate of acquisition. One concern

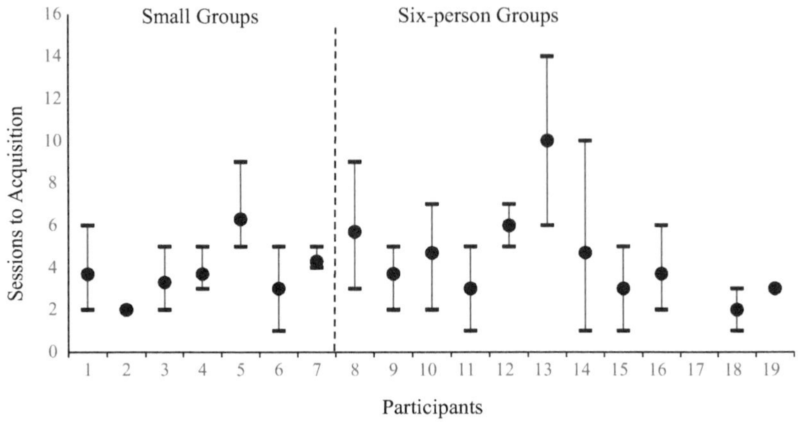

Figure 1 Number of sessions to acquisition of targeted skills for each participant. Mean number of sessions depicted by *closed circles*. Range depicted with *dashes*. Participants to the left of the *dashed line* were enrolled in the first two smaller group administrations of video-based group instruction. Participants to the right of the *dashed line* were enrolled in a revised iteration with six participants per group. Case 17 depicts a participant who never reached acquisition criteria.

about increasing group size was that participants may acquire skills, but at a slower pace. Fig. 1 depicts the mean number of sessions to skill acquisition, defined as 100% accuracy for an entire session, for participants in prior VGI studies as well as participants in the revised version with larger group sizes.

Overall, participants in larger groups demonstrated similar acquisition rates as participants in previous investigations, save for two cases. In one case, a participant in one of the groups did not meet the acquisition criterion and therefore is not represented in the figure. In a second case, the participant required 14 sessions to acquire the first skills, six sessions to acquire the second skills, and moved out of the district before we could assess acquisition for the third skills. Importantly, and similar to the previous administrations, participants in these larger groups showed a decrease in number of sessions to acquisition across targeted pairings, indicating that as participants learn from video models, they may become faster at learning from subsequent models.

The outcomes of the investigation with expanded group size suggest that VGI has potential to increase group size to six participants, which most schools are likely to prefer over a four-participant group. This was an important adjustment to build into the development process as it indicates a variable that could be altered by districts who implement VGI. All interventions are likely to be adapted by consumers with little guidance provided by intervention developers (Fixsen et al., 2005). The extent to which these adaptations maintain the core components of the intervention such that it can still be considered an empirically supported practice is likely to vary from one context to another. By building adaptations into the iterative development process, intervention developers can provide guidance to consumers about variables that can be altered without harming the validity of the original procedures.

3.2.5 Study 4: Addressing Issues With Generalization

Educators indicated during previous interviews that the skills acquired during VGI may not transfer to interactions with typically developing peers across the school environment. In alignment with teacher concerns, we observed several issues pertaining to generalization. Participants who had been through VGI during a prior academic year and following a summer vacation spent very little time around their typical peers even when placed in inclusive environments and did not demonstrate behaviors acquired during the previous year with typical peers despite having several opportunities to do so each day. There was a clear need to strengthen the intervention with a component that could support generalization. In addition, administrators had requested the implementation of peer-mediated intervention within the VGI procedures. Therefore, based on generalization issues and consumer feedback, we worked with school personnel to develop a complimentary peer-mediated intervention program that would train typically developing adolescents to interact with peers with disabilities, then bring the peers together with adolescents with disabilities to practice interacting in contrived and natural environments.

An experiment was conducted to examine whether bringing adolescents without disabilities into the VGI sessions would lead to generalization of skills targeted during VGI sessions. Novel video models were developed that incorporated the typical peers within the videos, then shown to participating adolescents with intellectual and developmental disabilities. In addition, after practicing skills with one another in a contrived setting, participants were taken to common social environments within the school (e.g., lunchroom, greenhouse) and provided with opportunities to practice the new social skills with typical peers. All participants acquired targeted skills, and more importantly, all skills generalized to novel peers in novel environments (MacFarland, Plavnick, & Kaid, 2014).

This last iteration of VGI was important in progressing to a full implementation stage (Fixsen et al., 2005) of the procedure following research activities. After observing the benefits of VGI for adolescents with ASD and other intellectual and developmental disabilities, as well as typically developing peers who had participated, the school district decided to incorporate peer-mediated social skills groups with VGI into its high school curricula. Peers were able to participate in the peer mediation program for elective credit in psychology, while adolescents with disabilities took the course for credit toward an alternative diploma. Three of the VGI facilitators within the school continued implementation of VGI during the subsequent academic year, when research was no longer being conducted, though a member of the research team provided some consultation. The intervention was then sustained by educators as the members of the research team faded completely out of the school.

3.3 Parallel Expansion

Simultaneous to our efforts to implement and test VGI within the school environment, we identified an additional area of need from consumers that we believed would be important for future adoption and implementation of VGI. Teachers had previously indicated the importance of additional videos, such that they could deliver a video modeling intervention for a broader array of social skills. School administrators had voiced a similar need, identifying the importance of social skill instruction for children across the autism spectrum. The school district wanted a single social skills approach that could be modified to support individualized instruction for a broader group of children.

Based on the demand for serving additional children, and simultaneous to carrying out the iterative development within schools, we sought to evaluate whether video modeling might be beneficial within a weekly social skills group format, often described in the literature for individuals with high-functioning ASD (e.g., Krasny, Williams, Provencal, & Ozonoff, 2003; Mitchell, Regehr, Reaume, & Feldman, 2010). Instead of daily administration with targeted and repeated practice of skills to mastery, groups met once a week and involved an overview of a specific social concept, modeling, and opportunities to practice with peers. The goals of the investigation were to examine whether participants performed better when skills were taught via video modeling compared to live modeling, assess whether instruction required the same number of facilitators, and evaluate whether children and families used video modeling content made available in an online learning management system.

Eleven participants with ASD between nine and 12 years of age were enrolled in two, 14-week social skills groups at a University Psychology Clinic. Five children participated in the first 14-week session and six in the second. All children had a community diagnosis of either autism or ASD. Participants attended a 1.5-h weekly session for 14 weeks. The curriculum was delivered from a procedural manual that was developed based on recommendations for best practices in group social skills instruction (Krasny et al., 2003; Mitchell et al., 2010). Group facilitators delivered either live modeling or video-enhanced sessions each week, with instructional conditions alternating in 3-week units.

For the video-enhanced condition only, children and their parents were provided with access to the video models after the lesson via an online learning management system that they could access at any time. The system included self-check questions that followed the video models to help the participant assess his or her understanding of the social scenarios using a multiple choice format and automated feedback. We measured the number of minutes a user logged into the system to interact with online instructional materials and the number of video models and self-checks each participant completed.

Although we found no clear differences in performance of targeted social skills during the video modeling and live modeling conditions, the video-enhanced social skills group sessions required fewer facilitators, likely for two reasons. First, because the model was provided by the video, a single facilitator could present instructional content to participants and a second facilitator was not needed to demonstrate social interactions. Second, facilitators were needed to support prosocial behavior and attending during live modeling groups. However, because participants attended better during video-enhanced sessions, these added facilitators were not necessary when videos were used for instruction. These findings are particularly relevant in school settings where a single service provider often administers social skills groups to multiple children with ASD.

Electronic tracking data from the video-enhanced sessions indicate participants used video materials outside the group sessions. Participants logged into the website a mean of 13.4 times (range, 2–20), accessed a mean of 63% of the content (range, 14%–89%), and spent a mean of 54.5 min on the site (range, 11–128 min). Despite high variability across participants, the site was accessed during weeks when video content was available and not during weeks it was not. This suggested an added value of video-enhanced instructional materials for teaching social skills to individuals with ASD. Although not a replacement for explicit social skill instruction, we are optimistic the data suggest an instructional website may have utility for participants and is worth evaluating its added value when included with more intensive social skill instruction, particularly when used with previously described VGI studies provided by school personnel on a more frequent basis.

4. SCHOOL-BASED INTERVENTION DEVELOPMENT

Conducting research during the development process of VGI raised questions that are likely consistent across a number of school-based research and development projects. For example, the process of creating an intervention that is efficacious, as well as usable and acceptable in school environments, creates the need for multiple rounds of testing and refinement. Although some alterations may be discovered during a short-term process of iteration (i.e., typical grant cycles), others may not be discovered until intervention developers attempt to assist in the sustained small-scale implementation of an intervention over an extended period of time. Because the implementation process requires adaptation (Fixsen et al., 2005), we believe that investigation of small-scale implementation cycles can help inform development of an intervention that can be sustained.

A unique feature associated with developing intervention packages is that components can be modified, recombined, or added to novel components to achieve optimal outcomes. There are several potential benefits to examining the effectiveness of isolated components or combinations of components before engaging in the more expensive task of examining the package as a whole (T. Smith et al., 2007). First, researchers can make refinements to ensure each component is highly effective and efficient. Second, continued evaluations of treatment components with individual cases clarify the boundaries of intervention effectiveness, thereby allowing intervention developers to build data-based modifications into the procedures. Modifications or "trouble-shooting procedures" can then be included within a developed manual, which is more likely to meet the needs of teachers and diverse student populations (Kasari & Smith, 2013).

One additional consideration to support adoption and sustained use of an intervention is a train the trainer model for preparation of interventionists. Although a training model was not formally examined with VGI, we included teachers who had implemented the intervention in training of educators who would implement in future iterations. Anecdotally, we believe this helped in the sustained implementation of the procedure as implementers had "in-house experts" who could provide technical assistance when needed. In addition, asking teachers to participate in training and to provide ongoing support lent credibility to the intervention. Part of community members' potential hesitation to adopt new interventions may relate to the belief that their situation is different than participants in initial studies (Cochran-Smith & Lytle, 1999). Therefore, by incorporating a colleague who has successfully implemented the intervention, it may be possible to reassure future interventionists that the protocol can be effective given their current circumstances. This may also help increase confidence of future interventionists as they may be more likely to equate their abilities to a peer who has been successful, as opposed to researchers.

5. CONCLUSION

Prior to more recent recommendations (Dingfelder & Mandell, 2011; Kasari & Smith, 2013), most intervention research in ASD followed a linear trajectory with an emphasis on answering the question "does the intervention work" (T. Smith et al., 2007). Such an approach may inadvertently facilitate the process of testing interventions in highly contrived environments and attempting to transport those interventions into school or other community settings. However, it may be important to first address questions such as "can and will service providers implement the intervention."

Dingfelder and Mandell (2011) present a theoretical series of questions that community service providers ask themselves before agreeing to implement an intervention. The first question asks about the existing evidence supporting how well the given program works. Researchers must be aware though that evidence in this case may not always refer to empirical evidence found in journal articles and may instead pertain to other sources, such as anecdotal evidence offered by colleagues. By alternating development and testing, our work with VGI has attempted to strike a balance between addressing the practical concerns and demands of teachers and providing sufficient evidence to convince teachers and administrators that the intervention is worth adopting and placing resources into implementing. The development of VGI involved several small experiments, the first conducted in a setting that approximated a school, and the rest within public schools.

Consumer feedback was frequently sought and helped shape the intervention into something that met the needs and wants of school administrators and teachers. These updated elements of VGI were then explicitly tested using rigorous single-case experimental designs. It is our hope that the interplay of ensuring intervention efficacy along with answering practical questions about implementation may form the foundation on which VGI proves to be an effective, usable, and sustainable intervention.

The development process of VGI involved an emphasis on designing an intervention that end users (i.e., educators) could feasibly implement and be willing to use. Intervention researchers will likely find it helpful to construct interventions in the environments where they envision future use. Doing so could optimize the intervention prior to rolling it out for effectiveness trials. Contextually based intervention development might therefore have greater benefits for consumers when compared to interventions developed in controlled university research settings.

ACKNOWLEDGMENTS

This research was supported in part by a grant from the Organization for Autism Research (#RC102238).

REFERENCES

Bellini, S., Peters, J. K., Benner, L., & Hopf, A. (2007). A meta-analysis of school-based social skills interventions for children with autism spectrum disorders. *Remedial and Special Education, 28*(3), 153–162. http://dx.doi.org/10.1177/07419325070280030401.

Berliner, D. C. (2002). Educational research: The hardest science of all. *Educational Researcher, 31*, 18–20. http://dx.doi.org/10.3102/0013189X031008018.

Blakely, C. H., Mayer, J. P., Gottschalk, R. G., Schmitt, N., Davidson, W. S., Roitman, D. B., & Emshoff, J. G. (1987). The fidelity-adaptation debate: Implications for the implementation of public sector social programs. *American Journal of Community Psychology, 15*(3), 253–268. http://dx.doi.org/10.1007/BF00922697.

Cochran-Smith, M., & Lytle, S. L. (1999). Relationships of knowledge and practice: Teacher learning in communities. *Review of Research in Education, 24*, 249–305. Retrieved from http://www.jstor.org/stable/1167272.

Cook, B., & Odom, S. L. (2013). Evidence-based practices and implementation science in special education. *Exceptional Children, 79*, 135–144.

Dingfelder, H. E., & Mandell, D. S. (2011). Bridging the research-to-practice gap in autism intervention: An application of diffusion of innovation theory. *Journal of Autism and Developmental Disorders, 41*(5), 597–609. http://dx.doi.org/10.1007/s10803-010-1081-0.

Durlak, J. A., & DuPre, E. P. (2008). Implementation matters: A review of research on the influence of implementation on program outcomes and the factors affecting implementation. *American Journal of Community Psychology, 41*(3–4), 327–350. http://dx.doi.org/10.1007/s10464-008-9165-0.

Fixsen, D. L., Blasé, K. A., Naoom, S. F., & Wallace, F. (2009). Core implementation components. *Research on Social Work Practice, 19*, 531–540. http://dx.doi.org/10.1177/1049731509335549.

Fixsen, D. K., Naoom, S. F., Blasé, K. A., Friedman, R. M., & Wallace, F. (2005). *Implementation research: A synthesis of the literature*. The National Implementation Research Network (FMHI Publication #121). Tampa, FL: University of South Florida, Louis de la Parte Florida Mental Health Institute.

Gillis, J. M., Callahan, E. H., & Romanczyk, R. G. (2011). Assessment of social behavior in children with autism: The development of the behavioral assessment of social interactions in young children. *Research in Autism Spectrum Disorders, 5*, 351–360. http://dx.doi.org/10.1016/j.rasd.2010.04.019.

Gresham, F. M., Sugai, G., & Horner, R. H. (2001). Interpreting outcomes of social skills training for students with high-incidence disabilities. *Teaching Exceptional Children, 67*, 331–334.

Howlin, P., Goode, S., Hutton, J., & Rutter, M. (2004). Adult outcome for children with autism. *Journal of Child Psyhology, 45*(2), 212–229.

Kasari, C., & Smith, T. (2013). Interventions in schools for children with autism spectrum disorder: Methods and recommendations. *Autism*. http://dx.doi.org/10.1177/1362361312470496.

Krasny, L., Williams, B. J., Provencal, S., & Ozonoff, S. (2003). Social skills interventions for the autism spectrum: Essential ingredients and a model curriculum. *Child and Adolescent Psychiatric Clinics, 12*, 107–122.

MacFarland, M. C., Plavnick, J. B., & Kaid, T. (May 2014). Using video-based and peer mediated instruction to facilitate generalization of social skills by adolescents with autism. In *Paper presented at the annual convention of the association for behavior analysis International, Chicago, IL*.

Mitchell, K., Regehr, K., Reaume, J., & Feldman, M. (2010). Group social skills training for adolescents with Asperger syndrome or high functioning autism. *Journal on Developmental Disabilities, 16*, 52–63.

Odom, S. L., Boyd, B. A., Hall, L. J., & Hume, K. (2010). Evaluation of comprehensive treatment models for individuals with autism spectrum disorders. *Journal of Autism and Developmental Disorders, 40*, 425–436. http://dx.doi.org/10.1007/s10803-009-0825-1.

Odom, S. L., Duda, M., Kucharczyk, S., Cox, A. W., & Stable, A. (2014). Applying an implementation science framework for adoption of a comprehensive program for students with ASD. *Remedial and Special Education, 35*, 123–132. http://dx.doi.org/10.1177/0741932513519826.

Orsmond, G. I., Krauss, M. W., & Seltzer, M. M. (2004). Peer relationships and social and recreational activities among adolescents and adults with autism. *Journal of Autism and Developmental Disorders, 34*, 245–256.

Plavnick, J. B., Kaid, T., & MacFarland, M. C. (2015). Effects of video-based group instruction on the acquisition of social skills by adolescents with autism. *Exceptional Children, 80*, 67–83.

Plavnick, J. B., Sam, A., Hume, K., & Odom, S. L. (2013). Effects of a school-based social skills training program for adolescents with autism spectrum disorder and intellectual disability. *Journal of Autism and Developmental Disorders, 45*, 2674–2690. http://dx.doi.org/10.1007/s10803-015-2434-5.

Rao, P. A., Beidel, D. C., & Murray, M. J. (2008). Social skills interventions for children with Asperger's syndrome or high-functioning autism: A review and recommendations. *Journal of Autism and Developmental Disorders, 38*(2), 353–361.

Rogers, E. M. (2003). *Diffusion of innovations* (5th ed.). New York: Free Press.

Rohrbach, L. A., Grana, R., Sussman, S., & Valente, T. W. (2006). Type II translation: Transporting prevention interventions from research to real-world settings. *Evaluation & the Health Professions, 29*, 302–333. http://dx.doi.org/10.1177/0163278706290408.

Seltzer, M. M., Shattuck, P., Abbeduto, L., & Greenberg, J. S. (2004). Trajectory of development in adolescents and adults with autism. *Mental Retardation and Developmental Disabilities Research Reviews, 10*, 234–247.

Slocum, T. A., Detrich, R., Wilczynski, S. M., Spencer, T. D., Lewis, T., & Wolfe, K. (2014). The evidence-based practice of applied behavior analysis. *Behavior Analyst, 37*, 41–56. http://dx.doi.org/10.1007/s40614-014-0005-2.

Smith, S. W., Daunic, A. P., & Taylor, G. G. (2007). Treatment fidelity in applied educational research: Expanding the adoption and application of measures to ensure evidence-based practice. *Education and Treatment of Children, 30*(4), 121–134. http://dx.doi.org/10.1353/etc.2007.0033.

Smith, T., Scahill, L., Dawson, G., Guthrie, D., Lord, C., Odom, S., ... Wagner, A. (2007). Designing research studies on psychosocial interventions in autism. *Journal of Autism and Developmental Disorders, 37*, 354–366. http://dx.doi.org/10.1007/s10803-006-0173-3.

Suhrheinrich, J., Stahmer, A. C., Reed, S., Schreibman, L., Reisinger, E., & Mandell, D. (2013). Implementation challenges in translating pivotal response training into community settings. *Journal of Autism and Developmental Disorders, 43*, 2970–2976. http://dx.doi.org/10.1007/s10803-013-1826-7.

Weinkauf, S. M., Zeug, N. M., Anderson, C. T., & Ala'i-Rosales, S. (2011). Evaluating the effectiveness of a comprehensive staff training package for behavioral interventions for children with autism. *Research in Autism Spectrum Disorders, 5*(2), 864–871. http://dx.doi.org/10.1016/j.rasd.2010.10.001.

Wood, J. J., McLeod, B. D., Klebanoff, S., & Brookman-Frazee, L. (2015). Toward the implementation of evidence-based interventions for youth with autism spectrum disorders in schools and community agencies. *Behavior Therapy, 46*, 83–95. http://dx.doi.org/10.1016/j.beth.2014.07.003.

FURTHER READING

Alessi, G. (1987). Generative strategies and teaching for generalization. *The Analysis of Verbal Behavior, 5*, 15–27.

American Psychiatric Association. (2013). *Diagnostic and statistical manual of mental disorders* (5th ed.). Arlington, VA: American Psychiatric Publishing.

Brugha, T. S., McManus, S., Bankart, J., Scott, F., Purdon, S., Smith, J., ... Meltzer, H. (2011). Epidemiology of autism spectrum disorders in adults in the community in England. *Archives of General Psychiatry, 68*, 459–465. http://dx.doi.org/10.1001/archgenpsychiatry.2011.38.

Chasson, G. S., Harris, G. E., & Neely, W. J. (2007). Cost comparison of early intensive behavioral intervention and special education for children with autism. *Journal of Child and Family Studies, 16*, 401–413. http://dx.doi.org/10.1007/s10826-006-9094-1.

Eldevik, S., Hastings, R. P., Hughes, J. C., Jahr, E., Eikeseth, S., & Cross, S. (2009). Meta-analysis of early intensive behavioral intervention for children with autism. *Journal of Clinical Child & Adolescent Psychology, 38*, 439–450. http://dx.doi.org/10.1080/15374410902851739.

Epstein, R. (1991). Skinner, creativity, and the problem of spontaneous behavior. *Psychological Science, 2*, 270–362. http://dx.doi.org/10.1111/j.1467-9280.1991.tb00168.x.

Gresham, F. M., & Lopez, M. F. (1996). Social validation: A unifying concept for school-based consultation research and practice. *School Psychology Quarterly, 11*, 204–227.

Howard, H. A., Ladew, P., & Pollack, E. G. (2009). *The national autism center's national standards project : Findings and conclusions*. Randolph, MA: National Autism Center.

Ingersoll, B. (2011). Early identification and treatment of social communication deficits in autism. *Current Directions in Psychological Science, 20*, 335–339.

Johnson, K., & Layng, T. V. J. (1994). The Morningside model of generative instruction. In R. Gardner, et al. (Eds.), *Behavior analysis in education: Focus on measurably superior instruction* (pp. 173–197). Pacific Grove, CA: Brooks.

McConnell, S. R. (2002). Interventions to facilitate social interaction for young children with autism: Review of available research and recommendations for educational intervention and future research. *Journal of Autism and Developmental Disorders, 32*, 351–372. http://dx.doi.org/10.1023/A:1020537805154.

Reichow, B., & Volkmar, F. R. (2010). Social skills interventions for individuals with autism: Evaluation for evidence-based practices within a best evidence synthesis framework. *Journal of Autism and Developmental Disorders, 40*(2), 149–166. http://dx.doi.org/10.1007/s10803-009-0842-0.

Shattuck, P. T., Narendorf, S. C., Cooper, B., Sterzing, P. R., Wagner, M., & Taylor, J. L. (2012). Postsecondary education and employment among youth with an autism spectrum disorder. *Pediatrics, 129*. http://dx.doi.org/10.1542/peds.2011-2864.

Steege, M. W., Mace, F. C., Perry, L., & Longenecker, H. (2007). Applied behavior analysis: Beyond discrete trial teaching. *Psychology in the Schools, 44*, 91–99. http://dx.doi.org/10.1002/pits.20208.

Strain, P. S., Shores, R. E., & Kerr, M. K. (1976). An experimental analysis of "spillover" effects on the social interaction of behaviorally handicapped preschool children. *Journal of Applied Behavior Analysis, 9*, 31–40. http://dx.doi.org/10.1901/jaba.1976.9-31.

Walton, K., & Ingersoll, B. (2013). Improving social skills in adolescents and adults with autism and severe to profound intellectual disability: A review of the literature. *Journal of Autism and Developmental Disorders, 43*, 594–615.

Zwaigenbaum, L., Bryson, S., Rogers, T., Roberts, W., Brian, J., & Szatmari, P. (2005). Behavioral manifestations of autism in the first year of life. *International Journal of Developmental Neuroscience, 23*, 143–152. http://dx.doi.org/10.1001/archgenpsychiatry.2011.38.

CHAPTER FIVE

The Promise and Practice of Peer Support Arrangements for Students With Intellectual and Developmental Disabilities

Erik W. Carter
Vanderbilt University, Nashville, TN, United States
E-mail: erik.carter@Vanderbilt.Edu

Contents

International Review of Research in Developmental Disabilities, Volume 52
ISSN 2211-6095
http://dx.doi.org/10.1016/bs.irrdd.2017.04.001

Abstract

This article addresses peer support arrangements as a promising and practical approach for supporting students with severe disabilities to access the myriad social and learning opportunities available within inclusive secondary school classrooms. My aim is to share some of what my colleagues and I have learned through the process of designing, delivering, and evaluating an intervention approach marked both by its efficacy and its feasibility. I begin by providing some context on secondary schooling to highlight both the complexities of supporting inclusive educational experiences and the enduring need for alternative support models. I then describe peer support arrangements and review research addressing the effectiveness of this intervention approach. Discussion then turns to the various ways in which core components of this intervention approach have evolved and been applied to support students. I conclude with recommendations for future research aimed at deepening our understanding of the application and impact of these interventions to support inclusive schooling for students with severe disabilities.

1. INTRODUCTION

Conversations about inclusive education have dominated discussions within the field of severe disabilities for more than four decades. Parents, educators, advocates, policymakers, researchers, and other stakeholders have all wrestled with—and vigorously debated—a progression of intriguing interrogatives. Why might inclusive educational experiences be important to pursue for students with severe disabilities? Where would such an education best be delivered? What are the essential elements of an inclusive education? How should such experiences be supported? In each of these four areas, old debates have endured and prior questions persist as contemporary concerns.

1.1 Why?

The rationale for inclusive education has been articulated in diverse and evolving ways. Early arguments emphasized the ways in which inclusive experiences might benefit students with severe disabilities. A host of anticipated advantages were advocated, including acquisition of critical social and communication skills, improvements in peer interactions, development of new relationships, enhanced learning opportunities, greater goal attainment, and higher expectations (e.g., Brown et al., 1979, 1983; Meyer, Peck, & Brown, 1991). Likewise, initial concerns about the potential detrimental impact of inclusive education on peers gradually gave way to exploration of how peers might also benefit from well-supported inclusion (e.g., Cushing & Kennedy, 1997; Kishi & Meyer, 1994; Peck, Donaldson, & Pezzoli, 1990). More recent conversations call for even broader consideration of how inclusive education might positively impact teachers, schools, and entire communities (e.g., Agran, Brown, Hughes, Quirk, & Ryndak, 2014; Carter, 2015).

1.2 Where?

From separate to neighborhood schools, from self-contained to shared classrooms—shifts in educational placement have emerged from longstanding debates about where students with severe disabilities should spend their school day. The 1980s and 1990s were marked by modest increases in the proportion of students with intellectual disability receiving at least some portion of their coursework within general education classes alongside their peers without similar disabilities (McLeskey, Henry, & Hodges, 1999; Williamson, McLeskey, Hoppey, & Rentz, 2006). More recent data, however, suggest some stagnation in these trends (Kurth, Morningstar, & Kozleski, 2015). Kleinert et al. (2015) reported that 12.6% of students with severe disabilities (i.e., those eligible for the alternate assessment) were served in separate schools, 70.7% in special education classrooms with some involvement in specials (e.g., art, music, physical education; less than 40% of the day), 8.9% in special education classrooms with some academic inclusion (e.g., math, science, reading; less than 40% of the day), and 7.0% in general education classes at least 40% of the day. Although most students with severe disabilities spend at least some time in general education classrooms, such participation continues to remain limited.

1.3 What?

Defining inclusion has been a particular challenge within the field of special education. Although sometimes used as a synonym for the general education classroom, a range of richer definitions have been proffered throughout the years. Most integrate elements of location, curricular focus, student and staff roles, the availability of supports, and social connections (e.g., Cushing, Carter, Clark, Wallis, & Kennedy, 2009; Ryndak, Jackson, & Billingsley, 2000). Early advocates placed an accent on the social aspects of the inclusive classroom; however, current conversations emphasize the importance of academic access and individualized goal attainment. Taken together, three areas of emphasis for students cut across contemporary descriptions of inclusive education—ensuring access to rigorous instruction, supporting relevant learning opportunities, and promoting relationships with peers (Carter & Draper, 2010).

1.4 How?

The question of how best to support students to access the social, academic, and other learning opportunities available within inclusive classrooms may be the most pressing of all current questions (Morningstar et al., 2016; Spooner, Dymond, Smith, & Kennedy, 2006). Myriad studies indicate the benefits so often attributed to inclusive education are not automatically accruing for students with severe disabilities (e.g., Carter, Sisco, Brown, Brickham, & Al-Khabbaz, 2008; Feldman, Carter, Asmus, & Brock, 2016; Soukup, Wehmeyer, Bashinski, & Bovaird, 2007). Indeed, the prevailing approaches used to support general education participation (i.e., individually assigned paraprofessionals) may ultimately fail to provide an educational experience characterized by rigor, relevance, and relationships.

This constellation of questions highlights just some of the pressing issues facing our field. We still need compelling data to determine whether our aspirations for inclusive education are being attained. In what ways are students, peers, staff, and schools actually benefitting from well-supported inclusive educational experiences? We still need strong studies that explore the experiences of students within general education classrooms. Does where students access the general education curriculum really matter? We still need a richer understanding of what marks an inclusive experience. What outcomes should we be pursuing within the context of the general education classroom? And we still need programmatic research that identifies effective pathways for supporting students with severe disabilities to participate fully and meaningfully in these settings. What are the best pathways for promoting access to rigorous instruction, relevant learning opportunities, and relationships with peers?

2. A FOCUS ON PEER SUPPORT ARRANGEMENTS

This article addresses peer support arrangements as a promising and practical approach for supporting students with severe disabilities to access the myriad social and learning opportunities available within inclusive secondary school classrooms. My aim is to share some of what my colleagues and I have learned through the process of designing, delivering, and evaluating an intervention approach marked by both efficacy and its feasibility. I begin by providing some context on secondary schooling to highlight both the complexities of supporting inclusive educational experiences and the enduring need for alternative support models. I then describe peer support arrangements and review research addressing the effectiveness of this intervention approach. Discussion then turns to the various ways in which core components of this intervention approach have evolved and been applied to support students. I conclude with recommendations for future research aimed at deepening our understanding of the application and impact of these interventions to support inclusive schooling for students with severe disabilities.

3. SECONDARY SCHOOL AS A UNIQUE CONTEXT FOR INTERVENTION

Special education research has been described as the "hardest of the hardest-to-do science" (Odom et al., 2005, p. 139). The configuration of secondary schools, the complexities of peer relationships during adolescence, the prevailing service delivery models, and the multifaceted needs of students with severe disabilities further compound the challenges associated with carrying out rigorous research and delivering inclusive practices as students get older.

3.1 Structure of Secondary School

As students enter middle and high school, the academic and social landscapes can change dramatically. Both the size and scope of secondary schools expand. For example, average student enrollment increases from 451 students in primary school to 575 students in middle school and 854 students in high school (U.S. Department of Education, 2011). The relative stability of elementary classroom settings gives way to students rotating through six to eight different classrooms each semester—each led by a different teacher, reflecting a divergent set of expectations and instructional approaches, involving a unique combination of classmates, and addressing a distinct curricular area. As the curriculum broadens to include a range of core academic, elective, vocational, and related arts courses, the content students are expected to master in each of these courses becomes more challenging.

As a result, the gap between what students with severe disabilities and their peers are expected to learn often widens. This diversity and rigor that characterizes secondary schooling highlights the necessity of intervention models that can be individualized when applied across learning contexts.

3.2 Complexities of Peer Relationships

Adolescence is a period when peer relationships elevate in importance and evolve in their focus (Brown & Larson, 2009; Lynch, Lerner, & Leventhal, 2013). Middle and high school students spend a growing proportion of their day in the company of peers and attribute increasingly more importance to these relationships across the grade span. In other words, the influence of peers becomes more prominent and students are concerned more about their reputations and the perceptions of others. Likewise, the loneliness ushered in by the absence of peer relationships may be more deeply felt (Gilmore & Cuskelly, 2014; Prinstein & Dodge, 2008). The ways students affiliate can also change. Dyadic interactions give way to group-based affiliations, and friendships increasingly form on the basis of shared interests, experiences, and values. All of these complexities provide the backdrop for peer interactions taking place in classrooms throughout the school day. This unique social context highlights the importance of ensuring intervention models are delivered in ways that foster valued social connections with peers and attend to the relationship dynamics that mark adolescence.

3.3 Prevailing Support Models

For most middle and high school students, academic instruction and support within their courses come primarily from the general education teacher and classmates. For students with severe disabilities, however, a divergent support model has remained dominant. The prevailing approach to supporting these students in inclusive classrooms has been the use of individually assigned adults (i.e., one-to-one assistance). Within this model, a paraprofessional provides direct and ongoing support to one or more students with severe disabilities enrolled in the class. Nationally, the number of full-time equivalent paraprofessionals working with students with disabilities far exceeds the number of certified special education teachers (415,781 vs. 339,383, respectively; U.S. Department of Education, 2016). Regional descriptive studies suggest many of these paraprofessionals are serving in individually assigned roles across school settings (e.g., Giangreco & Broer, 2005). For example, Carter, O'Rourke, Sisco, and Pelsue (2009) reported that 41% of paraprofessionals in their Wisconsin sample worked primarily in one-to-one contexts in high schools. Likewise, Fisher and Pleasants (2012) found that 36% of paraprofessionals in their Indiana sample spent part or all of their assignment providing one-to-one support. This widespread use of individually assigned support models has clear implications for how students are supported to access both learning and social opportunities available within inclusive classrooms. It also raises a host of concerns, particularly when sole instructional responsibility is delegated to the paraprofessionals and when the presence of an adult hinders academic engagement and social connections.

3.4 Diversity Among Students With Severe Disabilities

More than 634,000 students with intellectual disability, autism, and multiple disabilities between the ages of 12 and 21 attend public school in the United States (U.S. Department of Education, 2016). These adolescents comprise an extremely heterogeneous group of middle and high school students. Although those who have severe disabilities share in common their need for intensive and ongoing support, they also have highly individualized needs, strengths, and educational goals. In the area of communication, some are symbolic communicators, some are illocutionary communicators, and some are presymbolic communicators (Kearns, Towles-Reeves, Kleinert, Kleinert, & Thomas, 2011). In the area of social skills, they exhibit a wide range of strengths and challenges across subdomains (Lyons, Huber, Carter Chen, & Asmus, 2016). In the area of academics, some participate in assessments based on alternate academic achievement standards and others do not (Kearns et al.). And in the area of transition, students differ widely in their assessment profiles and planned postschool pathways (Carter, Brock, & Trainor, 2014; Shogren & Plotner, 2012). This considerable diversity emphasizes the importance of intervention approaches that can be personally tailored to address the individualized learning needs of participating students.

4. OVERVIEW OF PEER SUPPORT ARRANGEMENTS

Peer support arrangements are designed to provide access to inclusive educational experiences and foster social connections for adolescents with severe disabilities. This intervention approach involves equipping one or more same-age peers to provide ongoing academic- and social-related support to their classmate with severe disabilities within inclusive general education classes (Carter, Cushing, & Kennedy, 2009; Carter & Kennedy, 2006). Educational planning teams begin by identifying the supports a student with a severe disability will need to meaningfully access the learning and social opportunities available within a particular classroom. They further delineate which of these supports might come from peers, from the general education teacher, and from special education staff. Next, peers from within the same classroom are identified and invited to become involved in the intervention as "peer partners." Peers who agree to participate take part in an initial orientation session addressing their roles and responsibilities as a member of a peer group arrangement. Likewise, the paraprofessionals who will be facilitating the intervention are equipped to deliver it with attention both to fidelity and flexibility. When students begin working together, peer partners provide any number of contextually relevant supports. For example, they might encourage the student to contribute to class or group discussions, make introductions to other classmates, prompt appropriate use of augmentative or alternative communication (AAC) device, converse about common interests, or model how to respond to a question. Academically, peer partners might share class materials, collaborate on specific assignments, explain a key idea, or record an answer shared through AAC. Paraprofessionals (and classroom teachers) remain available to model relevant support strategies, provide constructive feedback, and offer encouragement as the students work collaboratively during various class activities. However, paraprofessionals gradually fade their direct support as participating students accrue experience and gain confidence working with one another. As appropriate, paraprofessionals may instead adopt a broader support role within a classroom, providing assistance to the general education teacher or supporting other students (Giangreco, 2010). Like other special education interventions, peer support arrangements are best implemented using a data-driven approach in which ongoing efforts are made to document the ways in which all students are impacted academically and socially by their involvement. Each of these intervention components—and the variations with which they might be implemented—will receive elaboration later in this article.

5. AVAILABLE INTERVENTION RESEARCH

Research examining the efficacy and social validity of peer support arrangements among adolescents with severe disabilities has spanned nearly two decades (see Table 1 for study information and primary research questions). Within this stream, my colleagues and I have carried out a program of research involving a series of descriptive, qualitative, and intervention studies aimed at further refining these support models to improve their impact, fidelity, and fit. In this section, I summarize some of what we—and others in the field—have learned about the impact of these interventions on participating students and staff.

5.1 Peer Interactions

Social interactions among students and their peer partners have been a primary focus of evaluation efforts. Indeed, almost every study addressing the outcomes of students with severe disabilities has included this as a central measure. Although somewhat varied definitions have been adopted across studies, a consistent finding is the substantial improvements in the occurrence of peer interaction when students with disabilities participate in peer support arrangements relative to alternative support models. Prior to intervention, students rarely or never interact with other classmates despite being enrolled in the same general education classroom. Different studies have provided more nuanced portraits of these interactions by also addressing the topics that students discuss with one another (social vs. task related; e.g., Biggs, Carter, & Gustafson, 2017; Carter, Asmus, et al., 2016; Carter, Moss, Hoffman, Chung, & Sisco, 2011; Carter, Sisco, Melekoglu, & Kurkowski, 2007; Chung & Carter, 2013), the social supports they exchange (e.g., Carter, Asmus, et al., 2016; Carter, Biggs, & Blustein, 2016; Carter et al., 2011; Shukla, Kennedy, & Cushing, 1999), the types of interactions (initiations or responses; e.g., Asmus et al., 2016; Biggs et al., 2017; Carter, Asmus, et al., 2016; Chung & Carter, 2013; Huber, Carter, Shaw, & Stankiewicz, in press), the appropriateness of interactions (e.g., Asmus et al., 2016), the communication modes students use (AAC, gestures, speech; e.g., Biggs et al., 2017; Carter et al., 2011; Chung & Carter, 2013), the persons with whom students interact (peer partners vs. other classmates; e.g., Asmus et al., 2016; Biggs et al., 2017; Carter, Cushing, Clark, & Kennedy, 2005; Carter et al., 2011, 2007; Chung & Carter, 2013), the occurrence of adult prompting (e.g., Chung & Carter, 2013), and indicators of interaction quality (e.g., Asmus et al., 2016; Carter, Asmus, et al., 2016; Carter et al., in press; Huber et al., in press). Three studies also anchored their interaction findings to normative comparisons of peers enrolled in the same classrooms (Asmus et al., 2016; Carter, Asmus, et al., 2016; Huber et al., in press). Such a point of reference is especially helpful

Table 1 Summary of Intervention Studies Evaluating Peer Support Arrangements in Secondary Schools

Study	Student/*Peer Partner* Demographics[a]	Setting/*Classes*	Student Outcomes Addressed	Primary Questions/ *Design*
Cushing and Kennedy (1997)	3 students: 2F, 1M; 3NR *3 peers: 1F, 2M; 3NR*	Middle school *English, health, science, social studies*	—	What are the effects of the intervention on peer partners? *ABAB, ABABAB, MBD across settings*
Shukla et al. (1998)	3 students: 2F, 1M; 2A, 1W *3 peers: 3M; 1A, 1 PI, 1W*	Middle school *English, math, piano*	Social interactions Active engagement	How does adult involvement influence the peer partner outcomes? How are students impacted by involvement in the intervention? *ABACABAC, ACABACAB*
Shukla et al. (1999)	3 students: 2F, 1M; 3NR *5 peers: 3F, 2M: 5NR*	Middle school *Art, social studies, math, industrial arts*	Social interactions Active engagement	What are the effects of the intervention relative to adult support models? *ABAB, ABABAB, BABAB*
Carter, Cushing, et al. (2005)	3 students: 1F, 2M; 3W *6 peers: 4F, 2M; 6W*	Middle/high school *English, science*	Curricular consistency Curricular contact Social interactions Quality of interactions	How does the number of peer partners (one vs. two) impact student outcomes? *ABAB, BABA*
Carter et al. (2007)	4 students: 3F, 1M; 1AA, 3W *4 peers: 2M, 2F; 4W*	High school *Biology, ceramics*	Social interactions Academic engagement	What are the effects of the intervention relative to adult support models? *Delayed MBD across participants*

Carter et al. (2011)	3 students: 1F, 2M; 2AA, 1W *6 peers: 5F, 1M; 1A, 1C, 4W*	High school *Ceramics, culinary arts*	Social interactions Academic engagement Support behaviors Peer and adult proximity	What are the effects of the intervention relative to adult support models? What supports do peer partners provide? How socially valid is the intervention? *MBD across participants*
Jimenez et al. (2012)	5 students: 2F, 3M; 5NR *6 peers: 5F, 1M; 6NR*	Middle school *Science*	Independent academic responses	What are the effects of the intervention on students and peer partners? *MBD across science units*
Chung and Carter (2013)	2 students: 1F, 1M; 1H, 1W *7 peers: 5F, 2M; 2H, 5W*	Middle school *Art, science, social studies, homeroom*	Social interactions AAC use Academic engagement Peer, adult, and AAC proximity	What are the effects of the intervention on students who use AAC? How socially valid is the intervention? *MBD across participants and settings*
Asmus et al. (2016)	3 students: 2F, 1M; 3W *10 peers: 7F, 3M; 10NR*	High school *Art, ceramics, social studies*	Social interactions Social contacts Peer proximity Friendships Academic engagement	What are the effects of the intervention relative to adult support models? How socially valid is the intervention? *Randomized trial*

(*Continued*)

Table 1 Summary of Intervention Studies Evaluating Peer Support Arrangements in Secondary Schools—cont'd

Study	Student/*Peer Partner* Demographics[a]	Setting/*Classes*	Student Outcomes Addressed	Primary Questions/ *Design*
Brock et al. (2016)	4 students: 1F, 3M; 1AA, 3W *10 peers: 8F, 2M; 1A, 1AA, 5H, 3W*	Middle school *Art, computer science*	Social interactions Individualized academic goals	Can a teacher-delivered training package improve paraprofessional implementation of the intervention? What are the effects of the intervention relative to adult support models? How socially valid is the intervention? *MBD across participants*
Brock and Carter (2016)	4 students: 2F, 2M; 1AA, 3W *11 peers: 7F, 4M; 1A, 2AA, 8W*	Middle school *Math, science*	Social interactions Academic engagement	Can a teacher-delivered training package improve paraprofessional implementation of the intervention? What are the effects of the intervention relative to adult support models? How socially valid is the intervention? *MBD across participants*

Carter, Asmus, et al. (2016)	51 students: 21F, 30M; 4A, 7AA, 2NA, 34W, 3O, 1 NR *106 peers: 73F, 33M; 4A, 13AA, 4H, 1NA, 81W, 3O*	High school *Art, band, chorus, computer technology, culinary arts, dance, digital arts, language arts, math, music, science, social studies, theater, wellness*	Social interactions Quality of interaction Peers contacted Individualized social goals Social skill ratings Friendships Support behaviors Academic engagement Individualized academic goals Class participation Peer and adult proximity Absence from the classroom	What are the effects of the intervention relative to adult support models? What supports do peer partners provide? How socially valid is the intervention? *Randomized trial*
Biggs et al. (2017)	4 students: 1F, 3M; 1AA, 3W *8 peers: 5F, 3M; 5AA, 3W*	Middle school *Foreign language, language arts, science, social studies*	Social interactions AAC use Support behaviors Academic engagement Peer, adult, and AAC proximity	What are the effects of the intervention involving collaborative planning relative to adult support models for students who use AAC? How socially valid is the intervention? *MBD across participants*

(Continued)

Table 1 Summary of Intervention Studies Evaluating Peer Support Arrangements in Secondary Schools—cont'd

Study	Student/*Peer Partner* Demographics[a]	Setting/*Classes*	Student Outcomes Addressed	Primary Questions/ *Design*
Huber et al. (in press)	3 students: 3M; 3W *8 peers: 2F, 4M, 2NR; 1H, 3W, 4NR*	High school *Art, nutrition, world history*	Social initiations and responses Interaction quality Academic engagement Peer and adult proximity	What are the effects of the intervention relative to adult support models? Can structural analyses be used to refine and improve the intervention? How socially valid is the intervention? *MBD across participants + multielement*
Carter et al. (in press)	4 students: 4M; 1AA, 3W *13 peers: 4F, 9M; 3AA, 1H, 9W*	High school *Business, math, physical education, science*	Social interactions and initiations Academic engagement Interaction quality Peer and adult proximity	What are the effects of the intervention without adult facilitation? How socially valid is the intervention? *Nonconcurrent MBD across participants*

A, Asian-American; *AA*, African-American; *AAC*, augmentative or alternative communication; *C*, Caribbean; *F*, female; *M*, male; *MBD*, multiple-baseline (or probe) design; *NA*, native American; *NR*, not reported; *O*, other; *PI*, Pacific Islander; *W*, white.

[a]Denotes only students participating in peer support arrangements.

when trying to determine what levels of interaction might be expected within or appropriate to a particular classroom. Finally, four of these studies captured the extent to which more sustained interactions (i.e., extended social contacts of 15 min or more) occur among students both during and after the semester (e.g., Asmus et al., 2016; Shukla, Kennedy, & Cushing, 1998; Shukla et al., 1999). Indeed, Carter, Asmus, et al. (2016) found that 40% of peer partners continued having social contacts one semester later.

5.2 Social and Communication Skills

The degree to which this intervention promotes social-related skill acquisition has received much less attention. In our randomized evaluation (Carter, Asmus, et al., 2016), we found that teacher ratings on a standardized social skills measure (i.e., Social Skills Improvement System) were not significant across groups of students of students who did and did not participate in a peer support arrangement. However, improvements in individualized social-related goals identified for the inclusive classroom were significantly better for students receiving the intervention. Likewise, we documented increases in AAC device use for all middle school students who worked alongside peer partners in Chung and Carter (2013); similar improvements were found for just one of four students in Biggs et al. (2017).

5.3 Peer Relationships

Inclusive education is often advocated as an avenue for fostering new friendships. Descriptively, peer support arrangements appear to be associated with the development of this important category, peer relationships. Interviews with or surveys of peer partners indicate most describe their new relationships as a friendship (Chung & Carter, 2013). These designations were reciprocated by students with severe disabilities in some studies (Asmus et al., 2016; Carter et al., 2011). For example, we found that 94% of students with disabilities said that their peer partners were friends, 96% of peer partners described their classmate with a severe disability as a friend, and educator-completed social network assessments aligned with these assertions (Carter, Asmus, et al., 2016). However, only two studies have experimentally examined the impact of peer support arrangements on friendship formation. In our recent pilot study (Asmus et al., 2016), we found that students were reported to have gained an average of 2.7 new friendships over the semester, relative to 1.7 new friendships for students without peer support arrangements. In a subsequent randomized trial in high schools

(Carter, Asmus, et al., 2016), we found that students in the intervention gained significantly more friends without disabilities than did students in the comparison group (2.25 vs. 0.60). Many of these friendships were quite durable. Among the 106 peer partners involved in this study, 40% were reported to have maintained their friendship one year later.

5.4 Academic Outcomes

The academic impact of these interventions also has received considerable attention. One rationale for introducing individually assigned paraprofessional supports into the inclusive classroom was the presumption that students with severe disabilities would require this ongoing support to participate fully in class activities. Thus, we have wondered whether students would become less engaged as they worked more closely with peer partners and adult proximity was reduced. Within this domain, most studies have relied on indirect measures of learning—primarily measures of academic engagement collected through direct observations (see Table 1). Some of these studies have differentiated between engagement in instructional activities that are or are not aligned with what other students are learning (e.g., Asmus et al., 2016; Carter, Cushing, et al., 2005; Carter, Hughes, Guth, & Copeland, 2005). Studies to date have reported divergent findings, ranging from no changes in academic engagement across conditions (e.g., Brock & Carter, 2016; Carter et al., 2011; Chung & Carter, 2013) to a mix of substantial improvements or comparable levels of engagement levels across conditions (e.g., Asmus et al., 2016; Biggs et al., 2017; Carter et al., 2007, in press; Huber et al., in press; Shukla et al., 1998, 1999). Other studies have shown that students gain more access to a range of academic supports when working with peer partners (Carter, Asmus, et al., 2016; Carter et al., 2011; Shukla et al., 1999). Measures of progress on more individualized academic goals have also been mixed. Findings from our randomized trial indicated some small, but nonsignificant, improvements in individualized academic goal progress within high school classrooms. In middle school classrooms, we found that three of four students demonstrated substantial progress on their individualized academic goals when working with peer partners (Brock, Biggs, Carter, Cattey, & Raley, 2016). Likewise, Jimenez, Browder, Spooner, and Dibiase (2012) documented increases in all five middle school students' use of science vocabulary words, pictures, word/picture match, and concept statements. Collectively, these findings suggest peer support arrangements are unlikely to hinder academic progress and may even enhance it.

Social validity. A persistent concern within the field of special education has been the degree to which research-based interventions can be carried out within ordinary schools and by actual educators. With few exceptions (e.g., Carter, Cushing, et al., 2005; Carter, Hughes, et al., 2005; Cushing & Kennedy, 1997; Shukla et al., 1998, 1999), most studies have examined key aspects of the social validity of peer support arrangements within general education classes. Respondents have included students with severe disabilities, peer partners, paraprofessionals, special educators, and general educators; no studies have solicited the views of parents or other classmates. The primary approaches included structured surveys and individual interviews; however, Jimenez et al. (2012) held a focus group with peer partners.

Although intervention implementation and participant perspectives have varied somewhat across studies, several themes are evident. When asked, most students with severe disabilities have indicated they enjoyed working with peer partners, considered them to be friends, and wanted to continue working together. Likewise, peer partners have expressed considerable confidence in their roles, described personal benefits, indicated they were not hindered in completing their own work, said they would recommend the role to others at their school, and wanted to assume this role again in the future. Overall, intervention facilitators (typically paraprofessionals) have considered the implementation time to be reasonable, reported they understood the procedures, expressed their motivation to use the intervention with other students, and indicated that participating students with and without disabilities benefited having involvement. Finally, general educators have been fairly positive about the time required to implement the intervention and its fit well within the inclusive classroom; however, their readiness to use the strategies in the future has been more tempered.

6. CONTRIBUTING FACTORS

Several aspects of this intervention approach may contribute to its impact (Biggs & Carter, 2017; Carter & Kennedy, 2006). First, peer support arrangements *establish shared activities* within general education classrooms. A robust finding throughout the severe disabilities literature is that presence alone does not ensure meaningful participation. In other words, enrollment in a general education classroom does not automatically translate into extensive social interactions and academic engagement. Both observational studies and the baseline phases of the intervention studies in Table 1 affirm the paucity of peer interactions and limited curricular access apart from intentional intervention (e.g., Carter, Hughes, et al., 2005; Carter, Sisco, Chung, & Stanton-Chapman, 2010; Hughes et al., 2012; Wehmeyer, Lattin, Lapp-Rincker, & Agran, 2003). For example, in one of our early observational studies involving 23 middle and high school students with intellectual disability and autism, we found that peer interactions and academic engagement were low and variable for most students, despite their presence in inclusive classes (Carter et al., 2008). In a more recent study involving 324 class-length observations of 108 inclusive high school classes, we found that students with severe disabilities were not in proximity to any other classmate during 58% of the class period (Feldman et al., 2016). Instead, we have seen students sitting next to a paraprofessional, working separately with other students with disabilities, or gone from the classroom (e.g., arriving late, leaving early). Peer support arrangements introduce planned and proximal opportunities for students with and without disabilities to work together throughout the semester.

Second, these interventions *increase social opportunities* for students with severe disabilities (Chung & Carter, 2013). Many middle and high school teachers rely extensively on instructional arrangements during which interactions among students are discouraged or diminished. Peer support arrangements establish interdependent activities that require students with and without severe disabilities to interact with one another, as well as introduce teacher-sanctioned interactions in the midst of lectures, whole-class discussions, and independent seatwork (Kennedy, 2001). Moreover, peer partners are encouraged and equipped to initiate conversations with their classmate with a severe disability, which likewise increases the probability that a student's communication attempts will be reinforced by peers (Biggs et al., 2017; Brock et al., 2016).

Third, peer support arrangements *promote curricular access* for students with severe disabilities (Carter & Kennedy, 2006). When students work primarily or exclusively with a paraprofessional, they may be less likely to participate in learning activities aligned with the rest of the students in the general education classroom. Whether a result of limited planning or insufficient preparation of paraprofessionals (Brock & Carter, 2013; Capizzi & DaFonte, 2012), this misalignment ultimately hinders curricular access. A collaboratively designed peer support plan articulates the ways a student will participate in the full range of learning activities taking place in a particular classroom, as well as the supports he or she will need to do so successfully. Ongoing work alongside peer partners serves to increase the response opportunities, corrective feedback, reinforcement, and individualized assistance the student with a disability receives. Likewise, peer partners stay attuned to whether the work their classmate is doing aligns with theirs and either advocate for or offer academic assistance in ways that pull the student into the curriculum.

Fourth, these interventions may *diminish stigma* by reducing the heavy reliance on specialized and adult-delivered supports (Carter, Biggs, et al., 2016; Giangreco, Doyle, & Suter, 2012). Students with severe disabilities spend a substantial proportion of classroom time in close physical proximity to individually assigned paraprofessionals. For example, we found the average time spent in close proximity to special education staff was 70% among middle school students who used AAC (Chung, Carter, & Sisco, 2012) and 50% among high school students with severe disabilities (Carter, Asmus, et al., 2016). During adolescence, the constant presence of an adult may make peers reluctant to initiate conversations or talk about topics unrelated to class (i.e., social conversations; Carter et al., 2008). Moreover, observing substantial differences in how students with disabilities are supported or the content they are learning may reinforce low expectations or negative perceptions among classmates.

Fifth, peer support arrangements *increase peer modeling*. For students with severe disabilities, thoughtfully selected peer partners model age- and context-appropriate social skills, demonstrate how to successfully navigate classroom expectations, and show students how to complete academic tasks. Indeed, peers may be the best experts on both local adolescent culture and valued conversational skills (Hughes et al., 1998). Such peer-delivered modeling facilitates observational learning (Bandura, 1977). This modeling also extends to classmates who are not directly involved in the intervention. Other students in the classroom may feel uncertain about how to interact with someone who uses a communication device, how to respond to unconventional behaviors, or how to work with someone who engages with the curriculum quite differently. Observing their peers responding to these situations in effective and enjoyable ways may increase their own confidence and willingness to get involved.

In summary, a peer support arrangement is an intervention approach that intentionally addresses a number of converging barriers that can coalesce to limit meaningful participation in inclusive secondary classrooms (Carter, Bottema-Beutel, & Brock, 2014).

7. CORE INTERVENTION COMPONENTS AND CONSIDERATIONS

Peer support arrangements are advocated as a flexible intervention approach that can be tailored to meet the individualized needs of a student with a disability and align with the unique expectations of a particular general education class. Although the studies we and others have conducted clearly incorporate a number of common intervention features, the ways in which individual components have been implemented have also varied within and across studies. A discussion of these components will serve to highlight both the flexibility of this intervention and potential areas for future study.

7.1 Collaborating on Intervention Design

An essential element of inclusion is the involvement of diverse team members who bring a breadth of perspectives and expertise to the planning of instruction and supports (Cook & Friend, 2010; Hunt, Soto, Maier, Mueller, & Goetz, 2002). In the same way, the design and delivery of peer support arrangements can benefit from the involvement of multiple stakeholders (Biggs & Carter, 2017; Mirenda, 2014). Example areas of potential contributions include the crafting of a written support plan, the choice of peer partners, the training of paraprofessionals and peer partners, the design of adaptations and modifications, or the collection and review of student data. Most evaluations of peer support arrangements, however, have involved only a narrow range of team members. For example, paraprofessionals and special educators typically work together to plan and implement the intervention, asking for limited input from the classroom teacher on the selection of peers or the appropriateness of the written plan (e.g., Carter, Asmus, et al., 2016; Huber et al., in press). In contrast, Biggs et al. (2017) elevated collaborative planning to a central component by involving paraprofessionals, special educators, paraprofessionals, parents, and speech–language pathologists in the development of intervention plans for middle school students with complex communication needs. Working together, the team crafted communication profiles for student, identified broad communication goals, delineated the ways in which peer partners might support those goals, developed a written support plan, and identified strategies that peer partners would need to be successful. Recognizing the logistical and structural challenges associated with effective collaboration in secondary schools, additional work is needed to identify multiple pathways through which key team members might contribute to the design and delivery of these interventions, as well as the way they enhance outcomes.

7.2 Equipping School Staff to Deliver Interventions

Early evaluations of peer support arrangements took place within the context of close collaborations among researchers and schools (Carter, Cushing, et al., 2005; Carter, Hughes, et al., 2005; Carter et al., 2007; Shukla et al., 1998, 1999). Researchers' involvement in the design and delivery of the intervention was more intensive and left open questions about whether similar outcomes would be obtained apart from such involvement. For example, university staff may have contributed to the development of the peer support plan, training of peer partners, or monitoring of students. To enable widespread implementation, staff from within the school community must be equipped to take responsibility for training and supporting paraprofessionals to facilitate peer support arrangements. Our more recent studies have examined implementation and outcomes when peer support arrangements are carried out by local school staff with limited external support. For example, Brock and Carter (2016) evaluated whether a teacher-delivered professional development package could enable paraprofessionals to implement peer support arrangements for four middle school students with severe disabilities. We found that special educators were able to deliver the training accurately, paraprofessionals were able to implement peer support arrangements with fidelity, and students experienced improved outcomes in their general education classrooms. Brock et al. (2016) extended these findings by also showing that paraprofessionals could readily learn to support peer partners in implementing targeted support strategies as they worked with their classmates with severe disabilities. Recognizing that special educators are likely the point persons for these particular interventions, avenues should be explored for embedding training on these interventions into preservice training programs and ongoing professional development. Presently, teachers may have limited confidence or experience implementing these types of peer-mediated interventions (Brock, Huber, Carter, Juarez, & Warren, 2014; Carter & Pesko, 2008).

7.3 Crafting Peer Support Plans

Ensuring students with severe disabilities access the myriad social and learning opportunities within a general education classroom requires intentional planning. The development of a written support plan serves to outline the individualized supports a student will receive from both peers and school staff across different aspects of the class. The structure for this plan has been refined over time and adapted to address particular purposes in some studies. The primary approach involves identifying (1) the main instructional contexts used throughout the semester (e.g., whole-group, lecture, small-group, labs, independent work, noninstructional transitions), (2) the ways in which a student with a severe disability will participate in these different class activities, (3) the specific supports that peer partners will provide during each of these activities, and (4) the ways in which the paraprofessional and general educator will assist the students to work together effectively (e.g., Carter, Asmus, et al., 2016; Carter, Biggs, et al., 2016; Carter et al., 2011, 2007). Chung and Carter (2013) adapted this approach to more explicitly address the social and communication needs of students who used AAC. Specifically, we worked with the paraprofessional to complete a planning tool that addressed how classmates without disabilities typically interacted with one another and actively participated during six segments of class (i.e., getting to class, when the teacher is leading the class, during small group work, during individual work, at the end of class) and then outlined how the student with a severe disabilities could interact and participate in similar ways using multiple communication modes. Biggs et al. (2017) adopted the primary planning structure, but incorporated specific communication goals that could be addressed during each segment of class and identified core vocabulary needed for each student's AAC device. Further refinements to these existing planning approaches might focus on more clearly delineating the academic modifications, accommodations, and instructional strategies needed to increase engagement with the general curriculum (Browder, Hudson, & Wood, 2014), as well as determining how plans might be revised throughout the semester in response to curricular changes.

7.4 Selecting Peer Partners

The prominent place of peers within these interventions highlights the importance of ensuring that selected peer partners are likely to be successful in and benefit from their roles. Surprisingly, considerations concerning the selection of these peers have received relatively little attention in the literature (Schaefer, Canella-Malone, & Carter, in press). In prior studies, different combinations of factors have been considered, including the extent to which peers have good attendance, work well with others, show an interest in or interact with the student, would be a positive model, or would benefit socially or academically from serving in this role. Each has been based primarily on the perceptions of school staff, and studies have not yet examined how these considerations are weighed or the impact of these choices on fidelity of implementation or student outcomes. In a few of these studies, the peer preferences of the student with a severe disability have been sought (Carter, Asmus, et al., 2016; Huber et al., in press); in most cases, paraprofessionals, special educators, and/or general educators make these decisions.

The primary purpose of the peer support arrangement should have some influence on the selection of peers. Ideally, educators are selecting peers who are well positioned to deliver key supports outlined in the written plan. When an intervention's accent is on fostering new friendships, however, the extent to which students have shared interests, common backgrounds, or overlapping activities outside of class may be worth considering. That is, friendships during adolescence are often characterized by similarity (Brown & Larson, 2009). Moreover, cultural considerations are also important here, as the choices individuals make about who they spend time with can be shaped by cultural, family, and other factors. Where there is an interest in impacting peer attitudes, school staff may want to consider inviting students whose prior experience with individuals with disabilities has been more limited. In other words, peers who volunteer for these roles tend to already have fairly accepting attitudes (Carter, Hughes, Copeland, & Breen, 2001; Shalev, Asmus, Carter, & Moss, 2016). Moving forward, much more attention should be given toward which selection considerations are most critical as well as to understand how such decisions impact the experiences and outcomes of students with severe disabilities.

7.5 Configuring the Intervention

Although peer-mediated interventions are advocated as a flexible approach for meeting the individualized needs of students with severe disabilities (Carter & Kennedy, 2006; Harris & Meltzer, 2015), relatively few configurations of peer support arrangements have been examined experimentally. For example, decisions must be made about how many peer partners to involve—too few can leave gaps in support during the class, too many could be disruptive or distracting. Carter, Cushing, et al. (2005) compared two intervention configurations (involving just one peer partner vs. involving two). We found that pairing two peer partners with one student resulted in higher rates of social interaction and comparable levels of academic engagement relative to involving just one peer partner. This triadic arrangement was also beneficial for peers, enabling them to share support responsibilities in flexible ways that allowed them to make adequate progress on their own work. Likewise, the involvement of school staff is important to consider. Shukla et al. (1998) examined the impact of adult facilitation on the active engagement of these peer partners. Huber et al. (in press) used structural analyses to identify those conditions under which peer support arrangements were most effective for three middle school students and then tailored the intervention accordingly. The revised intervention enhanced some outcomes for all participating students. Collectively, these studies suggest that different configurations of peer support arrangements can contribute to differential student outcomes.

As reflected throughout this section, any number of intervention elements could be adapted to meet the needs of a particular student (e.g., the choice of peer partners, the manner in which they are trained, the activities that students do together, the settings for intervention, the facilitation behaviors of staff). Future work should focus on identifying assessment-driven approaches for determining which configurations are most relevant and how they might be approached. For example, Huber and Carter (2016) identified 29 studies that incorporated some type of assessment to inform adaptations to peer-mediated interventions or the selection of student outcomes. These assessment approaches included formal and informal interviews, preference assessments, direct observations, questionnaires, document reviews, and structural analyses.

7.6 Nature of Supports

The supports that peer partners provide to their classmate with a severe disability can be influenced by multiple factors, including the content of the written peer support plan, the activities taking place in class, and the specific assistance that their classmate needs. Efforts to understand the nature of these supports and their impact have permeated this literature. Earlier studies examined the occurrence of social-related supports across six categories: access to others, help with decisions, information, material aid, companionship, emotional support, and greetings (e.g., Shukla et al., 1999). Subsequent studies adopted a broader list of supports across multiple areas, including academic-related (e.g., assisting with class assignments, prompting answers, reading aloud, assisting with notes, redirecting off-task behavior), social-related (e.g., reinforcing communication attempts, teaching social skills, encouraging interactions with classmates), and other supports (e.g., explaining or demonstrating class rules, helping the student self-manage behaviors; e.g., Carter, Asmus, et al., 2016; Carter, Biggs, et al., 2016; Carter et al., 2011). More recently, we have collected data on targeted peer support behaviors that have been explicitly addressed in peer partner training. For example, Brock et al. (2016) taught peer partners specific support strategies that matched to the individualized goals of the student whom they were supporting. All of the peers increased their use of these targeted strategies after training. Overall, available research suggests peer partners (1) exchange a wide variety of supports with their classmates, including supports not addressed in their training; (2) tend to implement social-related supports more often than academic-related supports; and (3) may be more likely to implement strategies when they are explicitly addressed in training.

7.7 Facilitating Collaborative Work and Peer Interactions

Although one recommended role for paraprofessionals within inclusive classrooms is the facilitation of shared work and social interactions among students (McDonnell & Jameson, 2014), a review of data collected across numerous baseline phases and comparison conditions indicates such facilitation infrequently or inconsistently takes place. Peer support arrangements shift paraprofessionals from an intensive to a supplemental role by fading physical proximity and increasing the use of facilitative behaviors. Although our early studies addressed facilitation anecdotally and assumed paraprofessionals were using the strategies they learned in their training (e.g., highlighting similarities among students, redirecting questions, modeling interactions, interpreting unusual behaviors; Causton-Theoharis & Malmgren, 2005), we soon began incorporating direct measures of the supports that these school staff provided as students worked together (e.g., Carter, Asmus, et al., 2016; Carter, Biggs, et al., 2016; Carter et al., 2011). More recently, we have refined these categories to improve our ability to document them reliably and to examine them experimentally. For example, Brock and Carter (2016) and Brock et al. (2016) arranged these paraprofessional supports into eight categories: prompting social interaction, reinforcing social interaction, providing information for social interaction, promoting academic support, reinforcing academic support, providing information for academic support, prompting proximity, and checking-in with peers. Both training and coaching led paraprofessionals to use these facilitation strategies more frequently.

7.8 Data-Based Decision Making

Regular reflection on the process and impact associated with peer support arrangement is essential within both research studies and implementation by ordinary practitioners. A data-driven approach to decision making is critical to understanding how this support model is being implemented and whether it is working well for all participants. In all of our studies, researchers rather than school staff have assumed primary responsibility for collecting and interpreting outcome, fidelity, and social validity data. The involvement of school staff in these areas has been limited largely to implementation. For example, several studies have provided checklists to paraprofessionals to self-monitor their facilitation of the intervention or fidelity of implementation (e.g., Asmus et al., 2016; Brock & Carter, 2016; Huber et al., in press). In addition, Carter, Asmus, et al. (2016) compared fidelity data collected by both research team members and school staff and found both to be adequately aligned. Moving forward, it will be important to identify effective ways of equipping school staff to deliver these interventions *and* adapt them in response to both formative and summative assessment data (Huber & Carter, 2016). Although data-based decision making is a core competency of special educators, application to this particular intervention approach is worthy of further exploration.

8. AVENUES FOR FUTURE RESEARCH

The considerable empirical attention allocated to peer support arrangements thus far has been encouraging and has contributed substantially to the field's understanding of the implementation and impact of this intervention. However, several aspects of these interventions warrant more focused attention. First, a host of measurement challenges still permeate this particular area of research. In terms of social outcomes, an emphasis on social interactions has eclipsed attention toward skill development and relationship formation. The extent to which students with severe disabilities are acquiring important social and communication skills that will generalize beyond the classroom and last over time remains uncertain but is important to discern. Likewise, documenting the emergence and growth of relationships among participating students and other classmates over time would benefit from much more sophisticated measurement approaches (cf., Bogenschutz et al., 2015). The extent to which these interventions contribute to a sense of belonging, membership, and acceptance has yet to be captured. In the area of academic outcomes, measurement must move from indicators of engagement toward documentation of goal attainment and learning (e.g., Jimenez et al., 2012). Although peer support arrangements can be considered an evidence-based practice for improving social outcomes, the same cannot be said for academic outcomes. Even as these measurement approaches are refined, difficult decisions will have to be made about which measures are most important to capture in a particular study and to document for a particular student. Such decisions are best answered by considering carefully (and collaboratively) the individualized goals of students and the outcomes that matter most in particular classroom.

Second, the adaptability of this intervention raises intriguing questions about what constitutes fidelity of implementation within the field of severe disabilities. Conversations about treatment fidelity within the broader field of special education often emphasize the importance of delivering interventions in prescribed ways and with consistency across students (Swanson, Wanzek, Haring, Ciullo, & McCulley, 2011). Yet, students with severe disabilities often require highly individualized interventions tailored to meet their unique needs, goals, and educational contexts. How do researchers navigate this balance between fidelity and individualization? What issues must be attended to when addressing efficacy and undertaking replication? In our more recent studies, we have strived to clearly delineate what we consider to be core and optional intervention components, to collect data addressing each of these areas, and to present our findings for readers to consider alongside both outcome and social validity data (e.g., Biggs et al., 2017; Carter, Asmus, et al., 2016; Huber et al., in press). Future work should explore alternative approaches, as well as work to identify which intervention components are truly critical and examine the parameters within which they can be implemented without diminishing impact.

Third, students with severe disabilities come from increasingly diverse backgrounds—ethnically, culturally, and linguistically. Across the studies listed in Table 1, 62% of participating students with severe disabilities were white, 26% were from other racial/ethnic backgrounds, and information was not reported for 12% of studies. How these interventions might be tailored with greater consideration of cultural and other relevant influences warrants much more attention in future studies. For example, how and with whom students choose to affiliate with their peers, the ways in which these interventions are introduced at a particular school, and the manner in which families are involved in supporting new relationships beyond the school day might each be areas in which these considerations have special relevance.

Fourth, advocates for inclusive education have long cited the potential benefits for classmates who learn alongside students with severe disabilities (Fisher, 1999; Peck et al., 1990). Most studies of peer support arrangements have descriptively addressed the impact on peer partners, primarily through end-of-experience surveys or interviews. Identified benefits have included changes in attitude toward students with disabilities, a stronger appreciation of diversity, unexpected personal growth, a deeper commitment to inclusion, the development of new advocacy skills, and the finding of lasting friendships. Articulating a stronger case for these interventions, however, will require speaking more directly to the ways participating peers—and perhaps their classmates—are impacted by their involvement. Such research will require more direct measures of peer impact and experimental designs capable of pinpointing the source of that impact (e.g., Cushing & Kennedy, 1997). Moreover, intervention components that might influence the experiences and outcomes of peers should also receive closer scrutiny. For example, how does the design of the initial peer training (e.g., length, content, and format) influence the confidence of peer partners and the benefits they accrue? In what ways does the ongoing support and facilitation that comes from paraprofessionals have an influence?

Fifth, conversations about inclusive education are no longer confined to elementary and secondary school classrooms. New postsecondary educational options are opening up for students with severe disabilities who are transitioning to adulthood. Indeed, nearly 250 colleges and universities have launched programs designed to support the inclusion of students with intellectual and developmental disabilities in all aspects of campus life. Many of these programs incorporate peer-mediated interventions into their support structures (e.g., Griffin, Mello, Glover, Carter, & Hodapp, 2016). To date, no efficacy studies have examined the extension of peer support arrangements to the postsecondary classroom. The adaptations required to make this approach work are intriguing, as college students may have much more capacity to provide complex supports and the greater independence students have on campus requires rethinking the roles of the intervention facilitator in the classroom. Application of the intervention to the college contexts clearly introduces a host of new complexities and opportunities.

Sixth, the paucity of longitudinal research is a continued concern—both in this area of research and throughout the field of severe disabilities (Ryndak, Alper, Hughes, & McDonnell, 2012). All but one of the studies addressed in this article spanned a single semester, leaving open important questions about the longer-term impact of these interventions. Carter, Asmus, et al. (2016) reported that 40% of peer partners had an extended social contact with their classmate with a severe disability during a 2-week window in the middle of the following semester and 43% remained friends. One year later, 16% of peer partners had an extended social contact during a 2-week window toward the middle of the semester, and 40% were said to be friends.

9. SUMMARY

Research on peer support arrangements has provided important insights into persistent and pressing questions about how best to support inclusive educational experiences for students with severe disabilities. Findings from this constellation of studies bolster arguments for why inclusive education can be so powerful for students with disabilities and their peers (why?). They illustrate the value of providing strong supports within general education classrooms (where?). They push for broader understandings of what it means to participate fully in these settings (what?). And they validate this intervention as an effective approach for promoting rigor, relevance, and relationships within inclusive contexts (how?). Although my colleagues and I are encouraged by what has been learned thus far, we also recognize that much more work is needed to flesh out fully meaningful pathways to inclusive education for all students (Morningstar et al., 2016). We invite new scholars to join us in further refining and evaluating this intervention to maximize its impact on students and its tractability in schools.

REFERENCES

Agran, M., Brown, F., Hughes, C., Quirk, C., & Ryndak, D. (2014). In *Equity and full participation for individuals with severe disabilities: A vision for the future*. Baltimore, MD: Brookes.

Asmus, J. A., Carter, E. W., Moss, C. K., Born, T. L., Vincent, L. B., Lloyd, B. P., & Chung, Y. (2016). Social outcomes and acceptability of two peer-mediated interventions for high school students with severe disabilities: A pilot study. *Inclusion, 4*, 194–214. http://dx.doi.org/10.1352/2326-6988-4.4.195.

Bandura, A. (1977). *Social learning theory*. Morristown, NJ: General Learning Press.

Biggs, E. E., & Carter, E. W. (2017). Supporting the social lives of students with intellectual disability. In M. L. Wehmeyer, & K. A. Shogren (Eds.), *Handbook of research-based practices for educating students with intellectual disability* (pp. 235–254). Oxford, UK: Routledge.

Biggs, E. E., Carter, E. W., & Gustafson, J. R. (2017). Efficacy of collaborative planning and peer support arrangements to increase peer interaction and AAC use in inclusive classrooms. *American Journal on Intellectual and Developmental Disabilities, 122*, 25–48. http://dx.doi.org/10.1352/1944-7558-122.1.25.

Bogenschutz, M., Amado, A., Smith, C., Carter, E. W., Copeland, M., … Walker, P. (2015). National goals for social inclusion for people with IDD. *Inclusion, 3*, 211–218. http://dx.doi.org/10.1352/2326-6988-3.4.211.

Brock, M. E., Biggs, E. E., Carter, E. W., Cattey, G., & Raley, K. (2016). Implementation and generalization of peer support arrangements for students with significant disabilities

in inclusive classrooms. *The Journal of Special Education, 49*, 221–232. http://dx.doi.org/10.1177/0022466915594368.
Brock, M. E., & Carter, E. W. (2013). A systematic review of paraprofessional-delivered interventions to improve outcomes for students with intellectual and developmental disabilities. *Research and Practice for Persons with Severe Disabilities, 38*, 211–221. http://dx.doi.org/10.1177/154079691303800401.
Brock, M. E., & Carter, E. W. (2016). Efficacy of teachers training paraprofessionals to implement peer support arrangements. *Exceptional Children, 82*, 354–371. http://dx.doi.org/10.1177/0014402915585564.
Brock, M. E., Huber, H. B., Carter, E. W., Juarez, A. P., & Warren, Z. E. (2014). Statewide assessment of professional development needs related to educating students with autism spectrum disorder. *Focus on Autism and Other Developmental Disabilities, 29*, 67–79. http://dx.doi.org/10.1177/1088357614522290.
Browder, D. M., Hudson, M. E., & Wood, L. (2014). Using principles of high quality instruction in the general education classroom to provide access to the general education curriculum. In J. McLeskey, N. L. Waldron, F. Spooner, & B. Algozzine (Eds.), *Handbook of effective inclusive schools: Research and practice* (pp. 339–351). New York, NY: Routledge.
Brown, L., Branston, M. B., Hamre-Nietupski, S., Johnson, F., Wilcox, B., & Gruenewald, L. (1979). A rationale for comprehensive longitudinal interactions between severely handicapped students and nonhandicapped students and other citizens. *AAESPH Review, 4*, 3–14. http://dx.doi.org/10.1177/154079697900400101.
Brown, L., Ford, A., Nisbet, J., Sweet, M., Donnellan, A., & Gruenewald, L. (1983). Opportunities available when severely handicapped students attend chronological age appropriate regular schools. *Journal of the Association for Persons with Severe Handicaps, 8*, 16–24. http://dx.doi.org/10.1177/154079698300800102.
Brown, B. B., & Larson, J. (2009). Peer relationships in adolescence. In R. M. Lerner, & L. Steinberg (Eds.), *Handbook of adolescent psychology* (3rd ed., pp. 74–103). Hoboken, NJ: John Wiley. http://dx.doi.org/10.1002/9780470479193.adlpsy002004.
Capizzi, A. M., & DaFonte, A. A. (2012). Supporting paraeducators through a collaborative classrooms support plan. *Focus on Exceptional Children, 44*(6), 1–6.
Carter, E. W. (2015). What matters most: Toward a future of flourishing. *TASH Connections, 41*(3), 10–20.
Carter, E. W., Asmus, J., Moss, C. K., Amirault, K. A., Biggs, E. E., Bolt, D., ... Wier, K. (2016). Randomized evaluation of peer supports arrangements to support the inclusion of high school students with severe disabilities. *Exceptional Children, 82*, 209–233. http://dx.doi.org/10.1177/0014402915598780.
Carter, E. W., Biggs, E. E., & Blustein, C. L. (2016). Relationships matter: Addressing stigma among students with intellectual disability and their peers. In K. Scior, & S. Werner (Eds.), *Intellectual disability and stigma: Stepping out from the margins* (pp. 149–164). London, UK: Palgrave McMillan.
Carter, E. W., Bottema-Beutel, K., & Brock, M. E. (2014). Social interactions and friendships. In M. Agran, F. Brown, C. Hughes, C. Quirk, & D. Ryndak (Eds.), *Equity and full participation for individuals with severe disabilities: A vision for the future* (pp. 197–216). Baltimore, MD: Brookes.
Carter, E. W., Brock, M. E., & Trainor, A. A. (2014). Transition assessment and planning for youth with severe intellectual and developmental disabilities. *The Journal of Special Education, 47*, 245–255. http://dx.doi.org/10.1177/0022466912456241.
Carter, E. W., Cushing, L. S., Clark, N. M., & Kennedy, C. H. (2005). Effects of peer support interventions on students' access to the general curriculum and social interactions. *Research and Practice for Persons with Severe Disabilities, 30*, 15–25. http://dx.doi.org/10.2511/rpsd.30.1.15.

Carter, E. W., Cushing, L. S., & Kennedy, C. H. (2009). *Peer support strategies: Improving all students' social lives and learning*. Baltimore, MD: Brookes.

Carter, E. W., & Draper, J. (2010). Making school matter: Supporting meaningful secondary experiences for adolescents who use AAC. In D. McNaughton, & D. R. Beukelman (Eds.), *Transition strategies for adolescents and young adults who use augmentative and alternative communication* (pp. 69–90). Baltimore, MD: Brookes Publishing.

Carter, E. W., Gustafson, J. R., Sreckovic, M. A., Steinbrenner, J. R. D., Pierce, N. P., Bord, A., ... Mullins, T. (in press). Efficacy of peer support interventions in general education classrooms for high school students with autism spectrum disorder. Remedial and Special Education. http://dx.doi.org/10.1177/0741932516672067.

Carter, E. W., Hughes, C., Copeland, S. R., & Breen, C. (2001). Differences between high school students who do and do not volunteer to participate in peer interaction programs. *Journal of the Association for Persons with Severe Handicaps, 26*, 229–239. http://dx.doi.org/10.2511/rpsd.26.4.229.

Carter, E. W., Hughes, C., Guth, C., & Copeland, S. R. (2005). Factors influencing social interaction among high school students with intellectual disabilities and their general education peers. *American Journal on Mental Retardation, 110*, 366–377. http://dx.doi.org/10.1352/0895-8017(2005)110[366:FISIAH]2.0.CO;2.

Carter, E. W., & Kennedy, C. H. (2006). Promoting access to the general curriculum using peer support strategies. *Research and Practice for Persons with Severe Disabilities, 31*, 284–292. http://dx.doi.org/10.1177/154079690603100402.

Carter, E. W., Moss, C. K., Hoffman, A., Chung, Y., & Sisco, L. G. (2011). Efficacy and social validity of peer support arrangements for adolescents with disabilities. *Exceptional Children, 78*, 107–125. http://dx.doi.org/10.1177/001440291107800107.

Carter, E. W., O'Rourke, L., Sisco, L. G., & Pelsue, D. (2009). Knowledge, responsibilities, and training needs of paraprofessionals in elementary and secondary schools. *Remedial and Special Education, 30*, 344–349. http://dx.doi.org/10.1177/0741932508324399.

Carter, E. W., & Pesko, M. J. (2008). Social validity of peer interaction intervention strategies in high school classrooms: Effectiveness, feasibility, and actual use. *Exceptionality, 16*, 156–173. http://dx.doi.org/10.1080/09362830802198427.

Carter, E. W., Sisco, L. G., Brown, L., Brickham, D., & Al-Khabbaz, Z. A. (2008). Peer interactions and academic engagement of youth with developmental disabilities in inclusive middle and high school classrooms. *American Journal on Mental Retardation, 113*, 479–494. http://dx.doi.org/10.1352/2008.113:479-494.

Carter, E. W., Sisco, L. G., Chung, Y., & Stanton-Chapman, T. (2010). Peer interactions of students with intellectual disabilities and/or autism: A map of the intervention literature. *Research and Practice for Persons with Severe Disabilities, 35*, 63–79. http://dx.doi.org/10.2511/rpsd.35.3-4.63.

Carter, E. W., Sisco, L. G., Melekoglu, M., & Kurkowski, C. (2007). Peer supports as an alternative to individually assigned paraprofessionals in inclusive high school classrooms. *Research and Practice for Persons with Severe Disabilities, 32*, 213–227. http://dx.doi.org/10.2511/rpsd.32.4.213.

Causton-Theoharis, J. N., & Malmgren, K. W. (2005). Increasing peer interactions for students with severe disabilities via paraprofessional training. *Exceptional Children, 71*, 431–444. http://dx.doi.org/10.1177/001440290507100403.

Chung, Y., & Carter, E. W. (2013). Promoting peer interactions in inclusive classrooms for students with speech-generating devices. *Research and Practice for Persons with Severe Disabilities, 32*, 94–109. http://dx.doi.org/10.2511/027494813807714492.

Chung, Y., Carter, E. W., & Sisco, L. G. (2012). Social interaction of students with severe disabilities who use augmentative and alternative communication in inclusive classrooms. *American Journal on Intellectual and Developmental Disabilities, 117*, 349–367. http://dx.doi.org/10.1352/1944-7558-117.5.349.

Cook, L., & Friend, M. (2010). The state of the art of collaboration on behalf of students with disabilities. *Journal of Educational and Psychological Consultation, 20*, 1–8. http://dx.doi.org/10.1080/10474410903535398.

Cushing, L. S., Carter, E. W., Clark, N. M., Wallis, T., & Kennedy, C. H. (2009). Evaluating inclusive educational practices for students with severe disabilities using the program quality measurement tool. *The Journal of Special Education, 42*, 194–208. http://dx.doi.org/10.1177/0022466907313352.

Cushing, L. S., & Kennedy, C. H. (1997). Academic effects of providing peer support in general education classrooms on students without disabilities. *Journal of Applied Behavior Analysis, 30*, 139–151. http://dx.doi.org/10.1901/jaba.1997.30-139.

Feldman, R., Carter, E. W., Asmus, J., & Brock, M. E. (2016). Presence, proximity, and peer interactions of adolescents with severe disabilities in general education classrooms. *Exceptional Children, 82*, 192–208. http://dx.doi.org/10.1177/0014402915585481.

Fisher, D. (1999). According to their peers: Inclusion as high school students see it. *Mental Retardation, 37*, 458–467. http://dx.doi.org/10.1352/0047-6765(1999)037<0458:ATTPIA>2.0.CO;2.

Fisher, M., & Pleasants, S. L. (2012). Roles, responsibilities, and concerns of paraeducators: Findings from a statewide survey. *Remedial and Special Education, 33*, 287–297. http://dx.doi.org/10.1177/0741932510397762.

Giangreco, M. F. (2010). One-to-one paraprofessionals for students with disabilities in inclusive classrooms: Is conventional wisdom wrong? *Intellectual and Developmental Disabilities, 48*, 1–13. http://dx.doi.org/10.1352/1934-9556-48.1.1.

Giangreco, M. F., & Broer, S. M. (2005). Questionable utilization of paraprofessionals in inclusive schools: Are we addressing symptoms or causes? *Focus on Autism and Other Developmental Disabilities, 20*, 10–26. http://dx.doi.org/10.1177/10883576050200010201.

Giangreco, M. F., Doyle, M. B., & Suter, J. C. (2012). Constructively responding to requests for paraprofessionals: We keep asking the wrong questions. *Remedial and Special Education, 33*, 362–373. http://dx.doi.org/10.1177/0741932511413472.

Gilmore, L., & Cuskelly, M. (2014). Vulnerability to loneliness in people with intellectual disability: An explanatory model. *Journal of Policy and Practice in Intellectual Disabilities, 11*, 192–199. http://dx.doi.org/10.1111/jppi.12089.

Griffin, M. M., Mello, M. P., Glover, C. A., Carter, E. W., & Hodapp, R. (2016). Supporting students with intellectual disability in postsecondary education: The motivations and experiences of peer mentors. *Inclusion, 4*, 75–88. http://dx.doi.org/10.1352/2326-6988-4.2.75.

Harris, K. R., & Meltzer, L. (2015). *The power of peers in the classroom: Enhancing learning and social skills*. Baltimore, MD: Brookes.

Huber, H. B., & Carter, E. W. (2016). Data-driven individualization in peer-mediated interventions for students with ASD: A literature review. *Review Journal of Autism and Developmental Disorders, 3*, 239–253. http://dx.doi.org/10.1007/s40489-016-0079-8.

Huber, H. B., Carter, E. W., Shaw, S. E., & Stankiewicz, K. C. Using structural analysis to inform peer support arrangements for high school students with severe disabilities. *American Journal on Intellectual and Developmental Disabilities* (in press).

Hughes, C., Kaplan, L., Berstein, R., Boykin, M., Reilly, C., Brigham, N., … Harvey, M. (2012). Increasing social interaction skills of secondary school students with autism and/or intellectual disability: A review of the literature. *Research and Practice for Persons with Severe Disabilities, 37*, 288–307. http://dx.doi.org/10.2511/027494813805327214.

Hughes, C., Lorden, S. W., Scott, S. V., Hwang, B., Derer, K. R., & Rodi, M. S. (1998). Identification and validation of critical conversational social skills. *Journal of Applied Behavior Analysis, 31*, 431–446. http://dx.doi.org/10.1901/jaba.1998.31-431.

Hunt, P., Soto, G., Maier, J., Mueller, E., & Goetz, L. (2002). Collaborative teaming to support students with augmentative and alternative communication needs in general education classrooms. *Augmentative and Alternative Communication, 18*, 20–35. http://dx.doi.org/10.1080/aac.18.1.20.35.

Jimenez, B. A., Browder, D. M., Spooner, F., & Dibiase, W. (2012). Inclusive inquiry science using peer-mediated embedded instruction for students with moderate intellectual disability. *Exceptional Children, 78*, 301–317. http://dx.doi.org/10.1177/001440291207800303.

Kearns, J. F., Towles-Reeves, E., Kleinert, H. L., Kleinert, J. O., & Thomas, M. K. (2011). Characteristics of and implications for students participating in alternate assessments based on alternate academic achievement standards. *The Journal of Special Education, 45*, 3–14. http://dx.doi.org/10.1177/0022466909344223.

Kennedy, C. H. (2001). Social interaction interventions for youth with severe disabilities should emphasize interdependence. *Mental Retardation and Developmental Disabilities Research Reviews*, 7, 122–127. http://dx.doi.org/10.1002/mrdd.1017.

Kishi, G. S., & Meyer, L. H. (1994). What children report and remember: A six-year follow-up of the effects of social con- tact between peers with and without severe disabilities. *Journal of The Association for Persons with Severe Handicaps, 19*, 277–289. http://dx.doi.org/10.1177/154079699401900404.

Kleinert, H., Towles-Reeves, E., Quenemoen, R., Thurlow, M., Fluegge, L., Weseman, L., & Kerbel, A. (2015). Where students with the most significant cognitive disabilities are taught: Implications for general curriculum access. *Exceptional Children, 81*, 312–329. http://dx.doi.org/10.1177/0014402914563697.

Kurth, J., Morningstar, M. E., & Kozleski, E. B. (2015). The persistence of highly restrictive special education placements for students with low-incidence disabilities. *Research and Practice for Persons with Severe Disabilities, 39*, 227–239. http://dx.doi.org/10.1177/1540796914555580.

Lynch, A. D., Lerner, R. M., & Leventhal, T. (2013). Adolescent academic achievement and school engagement: An examination of the role of school-wide peer culture. *Journal of Youth and Adolescence, 42*, 6–19. http://dx.doi.org/10.1007/s10964-012-9833-0.

Lyons, G. L., Huber, H. B., Carter, E. W., Chen, R., & Asmus, J. A. (2016). Assessing the social skills and problem behaviors of adolescents with severe disabilities enrolled in general education classes. *American Journal on Intellectual and Developmental Disabilities, 121*, 327–345. http://dx.doi.org/10.1352/1944-7558-121.4.327.

McDonnell, J., & Jameson, J. M. (2014). What are the roles of paraprofessionals in inclusive schools. In J. McLesky, N. L. Waldron, F. Spooner, & B. Algozzine (Eds.), *Handbook of effective inclusive schools: Research and practice* (pp. 94–106). New York, NY: Routledge.

McLeskey, J., Henry, D., & Hodges, D. (1999). Inclusion: What progress is being made across disability categories. *Teaching Exceptional Children, 31*(3), 60–64.

Meyer, L. H., Peck, C. A., & Brown, L. (1991). *Critical issues in the lives of people with severe disabilities*. Baltimore, MD: Paul H. Brookes.

Mirenda, P. (2014). Revisiting the mosaic of supports required for including people with severe intellectual or developmental disabilities in their communities. *Augmentative and Alternative Communication, 30*, 19–27. http://dx.doi.org/10.3109/07434618.2013.875590.

Morningstar, M. E., Allcock, H. C., White, J. M., Taub, D., Kurth, J. A., ... Jorgensen, C. M. (2016). Inclusive education national research advocacy agenda: A call to action. *Research and Practice for Persons with Severe Disabilities, 41*, 209–215. http://dx.doi.org/10.1177/1540796916650975.

Odom, S. L., Brantlinger, E., Gersten, R., Horner, R. H., Thompson, B., & Harris, K. R. (2005). Research in special education: Scientific methods and evidence-based practices. *Exceptional Children, 71*, 137–149. http://dx.doi.org/10.1177/001440290507100201.

Peck, C. A., Donaldson, J., & Pezzoli, M. (1990). Some benefits nonhandicapped adolescents perceive for themselves from their social relationships with peers who have severe handicaps. *Journal of the Association for Persons with Severe Handicaps, 15*, 241–249. http://dx.doi.org/10.2511/rpsd.29.2.135.

Prinstein, M. J., & Dodge, K. A. (2008). *Understanding peer influence in children and adolescents*. New York, NY: Guilford.

Ryndak, D. L., Alper, S., Hughes, C., & McDonnell, J. (2012). Documenting impact of educational contexts on long-term outcomes for students with severe disabilities. *Education and Training in Autism and Developmental Disabilities, 47*, 127–138.

Ryndak, D. L., Jackson, L., & Billingsley, F. (2000). Defining school inclusion for students with moderate to severe disabilities: What do the experts say? *Exceptionality, 8*, 101–116. http://dx.doi.org/10.1207/S15327035EX0802_2.

Schaefer, J. M., Canella-Malone, H. I., & Carter, E. W. The place of peers in peer-mediated interventions for students with intellectual disabilities. *Remedial and Special Education*. http://dx.doi.org/10.1177/0741932516629220. Advance online publication (in press).

Shalev, R. A., Asmus, J. M., Carter, E. W., & Moss, C. K. (2016). Attitudes of high school students toward their classmates with severe disabilities: A pilot study. *Journal of Developmental and Physical Disabilities, 28*, 523–538. http://dx.doi.org/10.1007/s10882-016-9489-x.

Shogren, K., & Plotner, A. (2012). Transition planning for students with intellectual disability, autism, or other disabilities: Data from the National Longitudinal Transition Study-2. *Intellectual and Developmental Disabilities, 50*, 16–30. http://dx.doi.org/10.1352/1934-9556-50.1.16.

Shukla, S., Kennedy, C. H., & Cushing, L. S. (1998). Adult influence on the participation of peers without disabilities in peer support programs. *Journal of Behavioral Education, 8*, 397–413. http://dx.doi.org/10.1023/A:1022801215119.

Shukla, S., Kennedy, C. H., & Cushing, L. S. (1999). Intermediate school students with severe disabilities: Supporting their social participation in general education classrooms. *Journal of Positive Behavior Interventions, 1*, 130–140. http://dx.doi.org/10.1177/109830079900100301.

Soukup, J. H., Wehmeyer, M. L., Bashinski, S. M., & Bovaird, J. A. (2007). Classroom variables and access to the general curriculum for students with disabilities. *Exceptional Children, 74*, 101–120. http://dx.doi.org/10.1177/001440290707400106.

Spooner, F., Dymond, S., Smith, A., & Kennedy, C. H. (2006). What we know and need to know about accessing the general curriculum for students with significant cognitive disabilities. *Research and Practice for Persons with Severe Disabilities, 31*, 277–283. http://dx.doi.org/10.1177/154079690603100401.

Swanson, E., Wanzek, J., Haring, C., Ciullo, S., & McCulley, L. (2011). Intervention fidelity in special and general education research journals. *The Journal of Special Education, 47*, 3–13. http://dx.doi.org/10.1177/0022466911419516.

U.S. Department of Education. (2011). Numbers and types of public elementary and secondary schools from the common core data. Available at https://nces.ed.gov.

U.S. Department of Education. (2016). *IDEA* Section 618 data products: State level data files. Available at https://www.ideadata.org.

Wehmeyer, M. L., Lattin, D. L., Lapp-Rincker, G., & Agran, M. (2003). Access to the general curriculum of middle school students with mental retardation: An observational study. *Remedial and Special Education, 24*, 262–272. http://dx.doi.org/10.1177/07419325030240050201.

Williamson, P., McLeskey, J., Hoppey, D., & Rentz, T. (2006). Educating students with mental retardation in general education classrooms. *Exceptional Children, 72*, 347–361. http://dx.doi.org/10.1177/001440290607200306.

CHAPTER SIX

Social Vulnerability in Williams Syndrome: A Tendency to Approach Strangers

Deborah M. Riby*[,1], Ellen Ridley*, Emma Lough*[,§], Mary Hanley*
*Durham University, Durham, United Kingdom
[§]Newcastle University, Newcastle upon Tyne, United Kingdom
[1]Corresponding author: E-mail: deborah.riby@durham.ac.uk

Contents

Abstract

In this paper we discuss the social profile associated with the developmental disorder, Williams syndrome (WS), and provide a specific focus on social vulnerability risk factors, such as social approach. To illustrate aspects of social vulnerability and social approach we introduce a case study on a 23-year old adult with WS and their parent. We link the core themes from an interview with the WS adult and their parent back to the existing literature. Finally, we discuss the challenges for future research in this area to inform both theory and intervention.

International Review of Research in Developmental Disabilities, Volume 52
ISSN 2211-6095
http://dx.doi.org/10.1016/bs.irrdd.2017.05.001

Successful social communication is critical to everyday interactions; not only is it essential that we can recognize familiar people within our environment, but we must also decipher a range of socio-communicative cues from the faces and bodies of the people that we interact with to adapt our own communication strategies. For example, is the person we are talking to angry or sad and how must we adapt our social interaction style accordingly? This type of social judgment occurs rapidly and automatically in typical development, but for some individuals with disorders of development this type of social skill is far harder, and difficulties deciphering social cues impact upon social interaction and communication on a daily basis.

Individuals of all ages with the neurodevelopmental disorder Williams syndrome (WS) can fall into this category, but as the social demands of daily functioning and independence increase through adolescence and into adulthood, these issues become even more crucial. In this review, we discuss the nature of the WS social profile before moving on to consider aspects of the social profile that might lead to enhanced social vulnerability for individuals (especially adolescents and adults) with the disorder. Social approach behaviors will be a particular focus due to their potential role as social vulnerability risk factors. We will give an example of social vulnerabilities from the insights of a parent and an adult with WS, relating to both real world and online interactions. Finally, we will consider areas for future investigation.

1. THE WILLIAMS SYNDROME SOCIAL PHENOTYPE

The social phenotype of WS has attracted significant research attention over the last two decades. Research throughout the 1990s had focused primarily on the cognitive profile of this relatively rare disorder, as characterized by a noticeable difference between relatively proficient language ability and more impaired spatial processing ability (e.g., Bellugi, Wang, & Jernigan, 1994), especially impaired spatial construction (Hoffman, Landau, & Pagani, 2003). This cognitive profile occurs against a backdrop of mild–moderate intellectual difficulties (Searcy et al., 2004) and the presence of peaks and valleys of ability led to a number of cognitive scientists utilizing the disorder as a model syndrome to explore modularity of mind (e.g., Bellugi, Adolphs, Cassady, & Chiles, 1999; Karmiloff-Smith, Klima, Bellugi, Grant, & Baron-Cohen, 1995; see also Levy & Herman, 2003). However, it soon became apparent that modularity of mind does not hold up for WS, as it is unlikely that any capacities develop "typically" and it is more likely that all aspects of cognition follow an atypical developmental trajectory (D'Souza & Karmiloff-Smith, 2011; Karmiloff-Smith, Brown, Grice, & Paterson, 2003).

At this point in the WS research timeline, relatively little systematic research had been conducted into the social phenotype of the disorder and a handful of studies focusing on face recognition ability led to the general consensus of relatively strong—and even the notion of "spared"—social functioning and face perception (e.g., Deruelle, Mancini, Livet, Casse-Perrot, & de Schonen, 1999). Indeed, face perception has often been used as a metric for social perception/social expertise. However, these studies on WS were predominantly restricted to very basic face recognition ability (e.g., using the Benton Face Recognition Task; Benton, 1980) and did not encapsulate the complexity of social information processing necessary to guide social communication (e.g., identity, eye gaze, basic expressions, and more subtle shifts of complex mental states, or complex socio-cognitive evaluations such as trustworthiness). Since this time there has been a wealth of research focused on more subtle components of face perception (including eye gaze and emotional expressions) and broader aspects of the social profile of WS. There is now a general consensus that social expertise, and certainly the development of face perception strategies, are far from "typical" in WS (e.g., Annaz, Karmiloff-Smith, Johnson, & Thomas, 2009; Karmiloff-Smith et al., 2004; Plesa-Skwerer, Faja, Schofield, Verbalis, & Tager-Flusberg, 2006).

There is considerable evidence to suggest that social functioning follows an atypical developmental pathway from a very early age and through adulthood in WS. It has been claimed a number of times that individuals with WS are outgoing, friendly, and gregarious individuals, who often display an "extreme" prosocial drive toward interactions with others, irrespective of their familiarity and across the developmental spectrum (e.g., Frigerio et al., 2006; Järvinen, Korenberg, & Bellugi, 2013; Jones et al., 2000). Evidence from young infants and toddlers suggests a desire to interact with others and an interest in attending to socially salient information. Jones et al. (2000) explored the development of the social functioning in WS with young infants (15–58 months of age) using the Parental Separation Task (Goldsmith & Rothbart, 1991). The frequency and intensity of affective responses were recorded when the infant was separated from, and subsequently reunited with, their parent. Young children with WS displayed an intense interest in other people (e.g., using direct eye contact) and exhibited fewer negative emotions compared to chronologically age-matched peers without WS. Such research has been used as an example of the "hypersocial" profile that is associated with WS and which emerges early in development and persists through to adulthood (Järvinen et al., 2013).

It could be questioned whether this hypersocial profile is "distinct" in WS (e.g., syndrome-specific) or whether this is an aspect of social behavior evident in any neurodevelopmental condition associated with intellectual impairment. Research has taken a cross-syndrome approach to explore this question and to understand any aspects of the social profile that might be specific to WS. Interestingly, it appears that the social phenotype of excessively friendly behavior is distinct even from other groups with intellectual impairments. For example, although individuals with WS and Down syndrome (DS) are often both considered to be social and friendly, it is the overfriendliness, social disinhibition, and difficulty forming and maintaining peer relationships seen in WS that distinguishes the social profile of these two groups (Dykens, 2000). Rosner, Hodapp, Fidler, Sagun, and Dykens (2004) compared to the social competence of individuals with WS, DS, and Prader–Willi syndrome across a very broad age range (4–49 years) using the Child's Behavior Checklist (Achenbach, 1991). Individuals with DS showed the highest overall social competence, followed by the WS and Prader–Willi groups, and age positively correlated with social competence for individuals with WS and DS. This suggests that although individuals with WS are more socially driven than individuals with DS (Doyle, Bellugi, Korenberg, & Graham, 2004; Jones et al., 2000), they are less socially competent. This distinction between wanting to engage in social interactions, and having the ability to understand social interactions, is crucial to the profile of social vulnerability that we see in WS compared to other developmental disorders.

2. SOCIAL MOTIVATION AND APPROACH

It is evident that across the developmental spectrum, many individuals with WS exhibit an extreme interest in social engagement and social disinhibition, irrespective of their social competence. For example, social motivation is one component of social function that appears to be less impaired in WS compared to other skills if we take basic information on interactions with others from measures such as the Social Responsiveness

Scale (SRS); (Constantinno & Gruber, 2005). Explicitly, a number of studies have used the SRS as a measure of social reciprocity in WS and across various studies there is relative consistency that as few as 13–17% of individuals with WS can be considered to show "normal" social behavior (e.g., across van der Fluit, Gaffrey, & Klein-Tasman, 2012; Klein-Tasman, Li-Barber, & Magargee, 2011; Lough, Rodgers, Janes, Little, & Riby, 2016; Riby, Hanley et al., 2014; Riby, Kirk, Hanley, & Riby, 2014). However, across these same studies, the subscale of social motivation shows the domain of least impairment of daily social functioning; for example, in research by van der Fluit et al. (2012) as many as 85% of the sample (n = 24; 8–15 year olds) were considered by parents to show social motivation within a "normal" range. Furthermore, in research by Klein-Tasman et al. this subscale was the domain of least impairment not only according to parents, but also according to teachers (SRS data from 82 parents and 49 teachers). This relative lack of impairment in social motivation seems to remain even in those with WS who are highly anxious (mean age 17 years; Riby, Hanley et al., 2014; Riby, Kirk et al., 2014).

There may, however, be a crucial issue with this evidence in that the SRS may not capture the subtle atypicalities of social motivation and social approach that are evident in WS. The measure was designed for use with individuals functioning on the autism spectrum and the social motivation subscale probes typical motivation and social withdrawal. The measure is not sufficiently fine grained to detect atypicalities of social motivation that are associated with increased approach and heightened motivation (e.g., the opposite of social withdrawal). More sensitive and "disorder-appropriate" measures of such behavior are crucial to advancing our understanding of this aspect of the WS social phenotype, especially given the potential role in social vulnerability.

One component of the hypersocial profile that we associate with WS (and potential vulnerability) is the desire to approach others, irrespective of their familiarity (Frigerio et al., 2006; Jones et al., 2000). Increased desire to interact with unfamiliar people is a particular risk factor in WS when combined with reduced intellectual capacity (Searcy et al., 2004) and difficulties understanding social communicative cues (e.g., trustworthiness; Martens, Hasinski, Andridge, & Cunningham, 2012). Studies of social approach behavior in WS have shown that individuals with WS would be more willing to approach both trustworthy and untrustworthy faces compared to typically developing (TD) individuals (Jones et al., 2000; see also Martens et al., 2012). Furthermore, Frigerio et al., (2006) found that it was faces that displayed positive emotions which individuals with WS rated as being most approachable, suggesting a link to emotion in social approach decisions (e.g., the amygdala hypothesis; Porter, Coltheart, & Langdon, 2007). However, these studies have relied on rating scales and the use of static face images in standard approach rating tasks (e.g., the Adolphs approach task used in a number of these studies, Adolphs, Tranel, & Damasio, 1998). More recently, research (including our own) has tried to use a range of different methods to explore components of typical/atypical social approach in WS, moving away from a reliance on rating scales, which might be particularly difficult for individuals to complete if they have intellectual difficulties, and using multiinformant responses. Given the importance of social approach behaviors in terms of social vulnerability this is an issue that warrants particular attention in WS.

Research using a video vignette task looked at the understanding of "stranger danger" and approach behaviors by individuals with WS and emphasized a lack of awareness that needs to be considered within their profile of approach and vulnerability (Riby, Kirk et al., 2014). Participants watched a short video extract of an interaction and listened to a story about that interaction before answering a number of questions about what was happening in the video. Only 27% of the answers given by individuals with WS (mean age 12 years) were deemed to show appropriate knowledge and awareness of issues relating to interactions with unfamiliar adults and aspects of stranger danger. This level of awareness was significantly lower than a matched group of much younger TD children of comparable verbal ability (mean age 7 years) who showed awareness in 60% of their answers.

Linking this "stranger danger" awareness to everyday social skills, those individuals with WS who showed less awareness of stranger danger were also those who experienced more peer relation difficulties and who generally showed less adequate prosocial behavior (as rated by their parents). Therefore, a lack of awareness of stranger danger may be a crucial component of the WS social phenotype that links directly to heightened vulnerability and is likely to come about from the constellation of difficulties individuals with WS experience when making appropriate social-cognitive judgments. Interestingly, there is preliminary evidence that some (but not all) adults with WS may benefit from stranger danger training programs, though further work in needed to support this suggestion and to devise thorough training packages (Fisher, 2014).

Our group has recently used a number of other paradigms to probe social approach behaviors, from parent reports to direct measures of social distance preference; all concluding the presence and importance of atypical social approach in the WS social phenotype. For example, using the aforementioned SRS measure, Lough, Flynn, and Riby (2015), Lough, Hanley et al. (2015) reported data from large samples of parents with sons/daughters from a wide age range with autism (n = 101; age range = 8−37), WS (n = 77; age range = 4−36) and those developing typically (n = 118; age range = 3−36). On the SRS there is one specific question that probes whether the individual "knows when he or she is too close to someone or is invading someone's space" and as well as the general social profile using the whole measure, this item was of specific interest. Parents reported that individuals with WS and autism were significantly more likely than those developing typically to invade the personal space of others. WS individuals were reported to have the least awareness of the personal space boundaries of others, even more than those with autism. Furthermore, relevant to consideration of age and social approach, there was no evidence that this issue changed with age in WS. This is evidence that social approach behavior may pose a risk for social vulnerability across development.

Parents can provide important insights into the everyday social behaviors of their sons/daughters with WS and in a study using parental interviews, several components of social difficulties were revealed (Lough, Rodgers et al., 2016). A qualitative semistructured interview approach can provide an opportunity to obtain rich data on social approach desires and this study involved interviews with 21 parents of individuals with WS around issues of social behavior and social approach, as well as the impact of social atypicalities. Using thematic analysis the interview transcripts revealed significant desires to interact with people and atypicalities of social approach that mirrored evidence from rating scale tasks (e.g., Jones et al., 2000), as well as a lack of awareness concerning strangers mirroring the previously mentioned task on stranger danger (e.g., Riby, Hanley et al., 2014; Riby, Kirk et al., 2014). It is crucial to emphasize, however, that there was vast heterogeneity reported between parents (and thus between individuals with WS) and this heterogeneity needs to be explored in future research to understand the potential mechanisms underlying differences in social approach and consequently differences in social vulnerability.

A final methodology that has recently been used to capture the nature of social approach in WS involves a "stop distance" task as a direct measure of how close the individual with WS stands to familiar and unfamiliar people (Lough, Flynn, & Riby, 2016). While this is an artificial approach situation, this direct measurement of social approach could be seen as more insightful than studies involving rating scales and the use of unfamiliar static adult faces as stimuli. This is also a more direct measure than using parent reports. The stop-distance paradigm has previously been used to assess preferred interpersonal distance (Kennedy, Glascher, Tyszka, & Adolphs, 2009) with various groups and individuals, such as those with amygdala damage. Compared to individuals who were developing typically, in this study those with WS showed a closer preferred interpersonal distance when approaching, and when being approached by, unfamiliar people. This group difference did not emerge for familiar people (e.g., interactions with their mother). So, the preferred interpersonal distance varied for the TD group based on familiarity, but not for the WS group. This is crucial because the individuals with WS did not modulate their preferred interpersonal distance in relation to the familiarity of the person they were interacting with, ringing bells with the notion that "everybody in the world is my friend" in WS (Doyle et al., 2004). Given that it is interactions with unfamiliar people that could be deemed as those that create social vulnerabilities, this issue is particularly important. Based on parent anecdotes during this study, it is highly likely that more natural social approach behaviors in everyday situations would reveal even more subtle atypicalities of social approach behaviors linked to decreased interpersonal distance. This remains an issue for further research.

This section of the review has emphasized that social approach behaviors are at the center of social vulnerability in WS. When these atypical social approach behaviors toward unfamiliar people are combined with reduced intellectual capacity (e.g., Searcy et al., 2004), increased and prolonged attention to faces (Riby & Hancock, 2008), and a range of difficulties interpreting social-perceptual and social-cognitive cues from others (e.g., Hanley, Riby, Caswell, Rooney, & Back, 2013; Plesa-Skwerer et al., 2006), it is easy to see how the individual with WS can be placed in a socially vulnerable situation. This vulnerability exists across the developmental spectrum and certainly does not decrease in adulthood (e.g., Davies, Udwin, & Howlin, 1998). It is more likely that the potential risk factors for vulnerability increase as independence becomes greater in adolescence and adulthood.

3. SOCIAL VULNERABILITY

The review so far brings us to a situation where individuals with WS are more prone to approach unfamiliar others and could be claimed to be in a socially vulnerable position. So, what is the evidence or understanding of vulnerability in this group? Vulnerability can mean that a person is in danger, highly susceptible to problems, and/or helpless (e.g., Grundy, 2006). Social vulnerability can be seen as a multifaceted term and we have previously taken the position that this describes "the disadvantages faced by an individual while he or she endeavours to survive as a productive member of society" (Jawaid et al., 2012, p. 335). It has been proposed that individuals with WS are at risk of experiencing abuse and victimization in their daily living because of a tendency for overly affectionate and socially outgoing behaviors shown by some individuals (e.g., hugging and kissing others; Davies et al., 1998), alongside their reduced understanding of appropriate social nuances. Davies et al. (1998) have gone further, beyond the social aspects of vulnerability, to claim that the risk for sexual abuse is heightened in adults with WS because of a lack of understanding of sexual matters.

In research by Fisher, Moskowitz, and Hodapp (2013), 79% of a sample of 38 young adults with WS reported some experience of victimization in their lifetime. In that study, parents of WS adults also reported that 37% had experienced teasing and the same proportion (37%) experienced theft or being tricked out of money. In fact, individuals with WS appear more at risk of vulnerability than those who have other developmental disorders such as autism or DS, partly because of relatively greater independence (Fisher et al., 2013). A great deal more research is required to understand this vulnerability and to provide appropriate evidence-based intervention or support. Furthermore, with societal changes to the nature of our interactions, such research also needs to consider vulnerability beyond face-to-face interactions (e.g., through online behaviors; Lough, Flynn et al., 2015). Recent research has emphasized that individuals with WS might be particularly vulnerable to online socially relevant risks, such as agreeing to meet an unfamiliar person they have interacted with on social media (see Lough & Fisher, 2016).

Picking up on this issue of online vulnerability, in a recent paper we discussed mapping real world vulnerability to that experienced online (Lough, Flynn et al., 2015, Lough, Hanley et al., 2015) because for individuals with WS who seek out social interactions, whilst simultaneously experiencing high levels of loneliness and anxiety during adulthood (e.g., Davies et al., 1998; Riby, Hanley et al., 2014; Riby, Kirk et al., 2014), it is clear why connecting with others via the Internet seems like an attractive prospect. We argued that if real world vulnerability can be used as a predictor for online vulnerability, then individuals with WS could face an elevated risk when interacting with others via the Internet (Lough & Fisher, 2016; Lough, Flynn et al., 2015, Lough, Hanley et al., 2015). Beyond these two recent studies of adults with WS, there is a lack of evidence concerning online behaviors of individuals with this developmental disorder, and indeed in individuals with other intellectual and developmental disabilities. But in this review, we finish with the insights from parents and an adult with WS to provide a case study revealing new data to highlight potential vulnerabilities both from real world social behaviors and online. We report a case study, which provides details about the online behavior of one adult with WS aged 23 years (pseudo name Grace). This is drawn from a semistructured interview carried out with the adult, and a separate interview with their parent. This interview did not involve discussion of victimization or abuse, but focused on the potential sources of vulnerability that might lead to victimization.

4. CASE STUDY OF REAL WORLD AND ONLINE SOCIAL VULNERABILITY IN AN ADULT WITH WILLIAMS SYNDROME

A semistructured parent interview was designed to address social behavior and Internet use in WS. There were four sections covering a general introduction, social profile, computer use, and risk and resilience (see Appendix for interview schedule). A case study approach was employed, and data were analyzed using thematic analysis, in line with the principles of Braun and Clarke (2006). The first section of the interview was developed to find out about their immediate family structure, as well as their daily routine and interests, and any particular strength they have. This information was designed to provide sufficient grounding to move on to the second section, which focused on the social profile. By understanding more about the social profile, the third section was able to address computer use and the online social persona. The final section was titled risk and resilience, which posed questions about vulnerability issues more directly. Note that this section did not explicitly include information on whether the individual had experienced victimization or abuse, but focused more broadly on potential risk factors for vulnerability (it was felt that there would be ethical issues with exploring sensitive and emotive personal experiences of victimization/abuse that were beyond the purpose of this case study). An adapted version of this interview schedule, focusing on the areas of social profile and computer use was implemented for the adult with WS.

It is worth noting that Grace is a 23-year old adult who has WS. The experiences and opinions that Grace and her mother provide in their interviews may be specific to Grace and may not generalize to all adults with WS, as is the case with this type of research endeavor. Indeed, parent interviews that we have previously conducted on social behaviors have emphasized vast individual variability, which feeds into heterogeneous social behaviors and variability in social vulnerability risk factors (see Lough, Rodgers et al., 2016).

The interviews were analyzed separately, and initial conceptualizations were developed from line-by-line coding. These codes were developed into themes, and the themes were applied back to the transcripts until saturation was reached. The same procedure was used to analyze the interview with the adult with WS. At this point, similarities and differences between the themes generated by the two accounts were analyzed, in an attempt to generate higher order themes, which encompassed the accounts given by both participants. Within each theme, the narratives were compared to produce results, which explored different perspectives on the same issues. Each transcript was coded for reliability. Cohen's kappa showed "substantial" agreement between coders for the account given by the adults with WS ($\kappa = 0.804$, $P < .001$) and "almost perfect" agreement between raters for themes generated from the parent account ($\kappa = 0.834$, $P < .001$; Viera & Garrett, 2005).

The results from a thematic analysis are shown in Fig. 1. These themes were generated from the responses given by the adult with WS and from the parent. Whilst the themes generated from the accounts given by Grace and her mother are the same, the content of these themes was different. The differences between the accounts are therefore highlighted in the following section, also linking some of these issues back to the literature presented previously in this manuscript.

4.1 Real World Social Behavior

The overarching themes that emerged from the interview were accounts of the hypersociable behavior displayed by Grace, mapping onto this widely

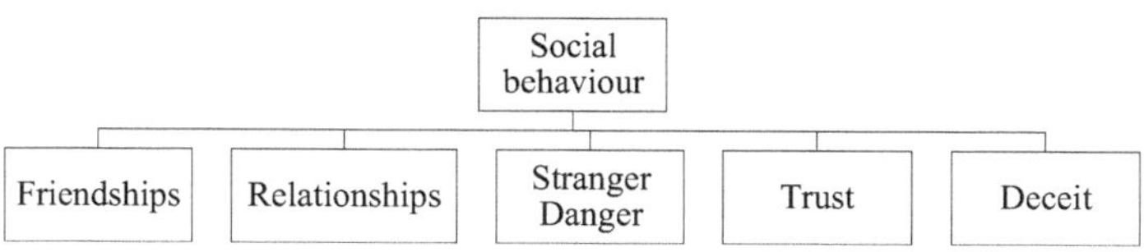

Figure 1 Thematic map of themes linked to social behavior.

reported aspect of the WS social phenotype (e.g., Doyle et al., 2004; Frigerio et al., 2006; Jones et al., 2000). The parent gave examples of her daughter's strong desire to interact with others, in contexts where it may not be considered socially acceptable, for example, "she will want to tell people who are serving her in shops one or two things about herself while she's getting the money out of her purse." These issues broadly link to aspects of social approach to unfamiliar people and social boundaries (or a lack thereof), as previously noted in this manuscript and the literature (e.g., Jones et al., 2000; Lough, Flynn et al., 2015, Lough, Hanley et al., 2015; Lough, Rodgers et al., 2016). The parent also noted how this behavior was a concern and impacted on her independence even during adulthood, for example, "we can't let her go out in the evenings really because she's just too small and vulnerable," again mapping onto issues of independence and social appropriateness of behavior previously highlighted by parents (Lough, Rodgers et al., 2016). The issues raised elsewhere in this chapter, which might form important vulnerability risk factors, therefore seem crucial in this case.

The theme of friendship emerged from both interviews, offering very different perspectives. It is worth noting that the literature emphasizes difficulty forming and maintaining friendships in WS, even in adulthood (e.g., Davies et al., 1998; Klein-Tasman et al., 2011; Udwin, 1990). Grace considered herself to have hundreds of close friends, whereas her parent identified these friendships as being more like acquaintances, for example, "to her, a friend is just someone who has smiled once at her." According to her parent, Grace struggles to form and maintain friendships, particularly with her peers. Grace seems to struggle to differentiate friendship behavior with relationship behavior, for example, she reported "I met a boy on my course and he accepted that I liked him actually he didn't run away from me so we were on and off for like 3 years we didn't kiss or hold hands or anything but he did really like me." Indeed, Grace has very blurred lines between strangers, friendships, and more serious relationships. This is something that has been evident throughout development, as noted by her mother "when she was little she liked walking and she would want to stop and talk to everybody coming the opposite direction," again emphasizing the "need" and "desire" to interact with others as reported elsewhere (e.g., Doyle et al., 2004). When Grace was asked what she does as an adult when she meets someone for the first time, she said "well for me I just say like 'hi, how are you?' And then when I see them again I say like 'I miss you' to ensure that they're ready for me because you know the friends that I see a lot give me cuddles and stuff and that shows me they've missed me. Then next time I give them a hug and literally I'm very emotional. One of my friends I had a big cry of joy with that I got to meet up with them again … it has been a long, long while, like a month." It is clear from this passage that strangers are quickly seen as friends by Grace, and there is a great deal of emotion attached to these "friendships." Furthermore, if Grace is willing to cuddle people so soon after meeting them this could be a potential vulnerability factor. The emotional content of this passage, and the emotionally driven behaviors that Grace emphasizes, link directly to reports of heightened emotional responses and empathy among individuals with WS (e.g., Fidler, Hepburn, Most, Philofsky, & Rogers, 2007; Plesa Skwerer et al., 2016).

Related to situations of vulnerability, the issues of trust and deceit emerged from the interviews. Research involving adults has previously suggested a link between trust evaluations and social approach in WS (e.g., see Martens et al., 2012) though research has also suggested that adults with WS can detect lies and appropriately evaluate trust from faces on this basis (Ng, Fillet, De Witt, Heyman, & Bellugi, 2015). When Grace was asked how she knew if she could trust someone, she replied "well it's like if they show it to me if they act as though they love me and comfort me … like my friends said to me 'we'll look after you' and things like that and that showed me I could trust them so saying nice things to me." This definition of trust seems entwined with basic kindness and her mother noted "I don't think she has the ability there at all to make these trust judgements" indeed she went on to emphasize that "if someone sophisticated lied to her I don't think she would have a clue. I think she would be very vulnerable to grooming and that's still a concern." Therefore these insights do not suggest that Grace is as good at accurately making trustworthiness evaluations as might be expected based on research by Ng et al. (2015).

4.2 Internet Interactions

A second thematic diagram (see Fig. 2) was produced to depict themes which came from the discussion of Internet use. Responses from the adult

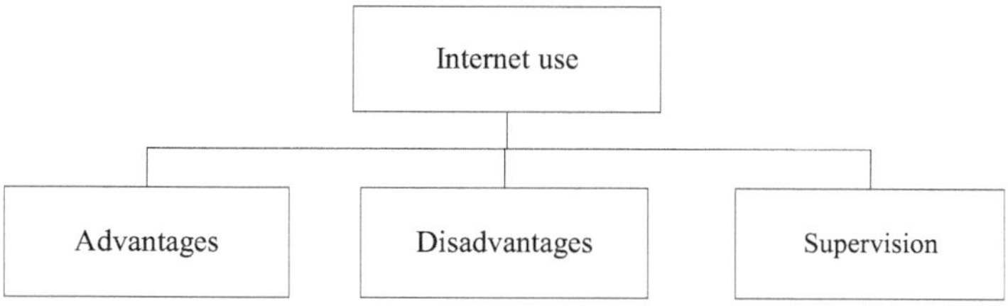

Figure 2 Thematic map summarizing the key themes on Internet use.

with WS and her parent were used to generate these themes. Grace uses the Internet for a variety of reasons, and her mother reported that now she is an adult, she spends a great deal of time on the computer. This maps on to recent research that reports frequent use of the Internet and social media by adults with WS (Lough & Fisher, 2016), although it goes against research on individuals with general intellectual and developmental disabilities which suggests that this group is less likely to use social networking sites (68% vs. 82% for those without additional needs; Wells & Mitchell, 2013). Grace emphasized "I go on Facebook. I go on YouTube and watch music videos and watch videos of things like washing machines and proposals you know nice little things." There is clearly the opportunity for Grace to interact with others through her Internet use, for example, via Facebook and interestingly, her broad definition of friendship extends to online social networking, as Grace said she has over "1000 friends on Facebook". Her hypersociability, and difficulties understanding social nuances, also seem to be evident in her virtual friendships as illustrated in the following quote from Grace:

> *"When people want space or when people want me to end the friendship they tell me. I've ended a few friendships over Facebook because they weren't wanting me as a friend they weren't wanting my love they just didn't see how I felt. They messaged me saying that loads and loads and loads of times so I ended the friendship. I've only started to speak to a few of them again properly now, because this time they're ready they weren't ready last time, I just wish they could have seen it. I just know they're ready. They need to understand that it's just me trying to show love to them. My mum says if they don't want me, I have to let them go, but you know I'm a special needs person so I can't do that it's very hard."*

Grace was keen to stress the advantages of the Internet for her, highlighting that it opens up new methods of social interaction and communication, for example, "I can talk to friends I don't get to see at all. So like I can see their face, I can see what's happening in their life, I can see how I can help them out ... Facebook has opened up so many new things, like before Facebook I was ringing up people's houses and sometimes people don't answer the house phone and now I can message them without having to ring them." This potential positive impact was something that was also emphasized by her mother. These online friendships give Grace some of the social stimulation that she seeks, for example, "it gives her proxy friendships really when friendship is difficult elsewhere." Having noted previously that the literature highlights problems with friendships in WS this is an important avenue for social engagement (e.g., Udwin, 1990).

However, there are also disadvantages to this Internet use and that was acknowledged by both Grace and her mother, although they saw the types and severity of these disadvantages very differently. The focus for Grace was on being tricked by scam e-mails, for example, "little things like they might trick you and some things like e-mails that come up that you shouldn't open but you want to open." Although Grace may seem aware of this specific type of risk, her mother emphasizes that her Internet use has the ability to heighten her vulnerabilities and safety concerns. For example, her mother emphasized that "because she has Facebook on her phone, ... she put as her status I'm going to this place, who wants to meet me, and there was no-one accompanying her so I think she made herself very vulnerable saying she would be in a certain café at a certain time and 1000 people know that she's there and waiting to talk, it's very, very open to abuse." Furthermore, while her mother said that Grace is likely to talk to her about things that had upset her online, she also talks to people online about things that had upset her in the real world. This lack of social boundaries is something that seems to be present for Grace both offline and online and her mother emphasizes that the vulnerability experienced by Grace in her daily life is very similar to that she experiences online, for example, "it's the same really. Except it's a bit more difficult online because it's there in the home isn't it, you can't lock the door and it's gone." These issues are important because research by Lough and Fisher (2016) has emphasized that individuals with WS are especially prone to socially oriented risky behavior when online, even more than nonsocial risks; for example, agreeing to meet unfamiliar people they have interacted with online.

In terms of supervision online, Grace's mother tries to set rules to keep her safe, but acknowledges that they are difficult to enforce, though Grace does view her mother's input in a positive way, seeing her as being helpful rather than overprotective.

4.3 Conclusions

The aim of this case study was to gain an insight into one adult with WS, from her perspective and from the perspective of her mother. Findings from the case study interviews identified key themes relating to social behavior and Internet use. Hypersociability and a lack of stranger danger awareness were apparent across these themes, both in the real world and online. These issues map on to make up the areas already highlighted in this paper, and emphasize the heightened vulnerability that may result as a consequence of such behaviors. The case study goes some way in emphasizing that in society today we need to acknowledge the varied routes to socialization used by individuals with intellectual difficulties such as WS, and feed this into our intervention and support packages, as well as our conceptualization of social vulnerability and the expression of the social phenotype. Although this interview did not focus on abuse or victimization, another future avenue of investigation may be the potential for some of these vulnerability risk factors to lead directly to victimization.

5. NEXT STEPS AND CONCLUSIONS

This chapter has narrowly focused on individuals with WS so that it is possible to provide in-depth understanding of social behaviors and potential vulnerabilities in this group. However, in future research we should also look at the evidence from other intellectual and developmental disabilities to see whether these characteristics are generalized, or more specific to WS. Cross-syndrome approaches are particularly insightful for understanding syndrome-specificity of this nature and are crucial for developing theories of social behavior. Parental reports from adolescents and adults with WS, DS, and autism have suggested that those with WS are at heightened risk for perceived vulnerability compared to these other developmental disorder groups (Fisher et al., 2013). However, there is currently a dearth of research systematically comparing these issues across disorders and throughout development, or providing core, sensitive measures that can reliabily be applied across developmental conditions.

There has been a vast expansion in our understanding of the social phenotype of WS over the last 20 years and we have moved a long way from the conceptualization of "intact" social skills, or that social behaviors are always a "strength." In this manuscript, we have detailed the literature on social behaviors, with a specific focus on social approach, to lay the foundation for why individuals with WS might be at risk of heightened social vulnerability. We have brought these issues to life with use of a case study from a 23-year old adult with WS and their parent. The variety of methodologies used to study social approach and vulnerabilities has grown exponentially over the last decade and researchers need to grasp the opportunity to utilize multimethods and multiinformant insights to understand the components of social behavior and vulnerability in this group. While some previous studies have emphasized agreement between parents and teachers in terms of social behaviors in WS (e.g., see Klein-Tasman et al., 2011), other studies have emphasized that parent and self-reports of social skills vary, especially around friendships (e.g., Freeman, Williams, Farran, & Brown, 2010) as supported by the current case study. Importantly, individuals with WS might fail to recognize their own social difficulties, which may lead them to be vulnerable to exploitation and therefore insights from a variety of sources is important (Lough & Fisher, 2016). As noted above, before it is possible to advance a multimethods and multiinformant approach we need suitable methods of measurement for the constructs we are studying here; for example, aspects of vulnerability, approach, etc., that can be utilized to gather different perspectives from different informants, and for different developmental disorder groups. We are not currently at this stage and future research should focus on this measurement issue to really advance our understanding across disorders.

While this manuscript has not taken a theoretical stance in the discussion of social behaviors or vulnerabilities, there is a great deal of work still to do in terms of a theoretical perspective, especially weighting up the role of frontal lobe functioning (e.g., see Little et al., 2013), the involvement of the amygdala (e.g., Porter et al., 2007) and advancing our understanding of genetic contributions to the WS social phenotype (e.g., see Järvinen & Bellugi, 2013; Järvinen et al., 2013). At present the debate concerning a theory of social behavior in WS revolves around these issues, with evidence providing a role for the amygdala, the frontal lobes, and genetic contributions. It is important that in the future we have a clear understanding of the mechanisms underlying social behaviors in this group to feed this into our theories of the disorder, into consideration of intervention approaches, and to be able to understand their potential role in vulnerability risks in WS.

It is indeed the case that many individuals with WS strive for emotional connectedness and social interactions, but this does not mean that they are always good at understanding social signals and using them to adapt and guide their own behaviors accordingly. There are a wide range of subtle but impactful atypicalities within the social phenotype of WS as illustrated in this manuscript, and there is still a great deal more research needed to understand some of the mechanisms underlying those social atypicalities; for example, atypicalities of social attention, of social approach/motivations, and of heightened vulnerability. These social atypicalities and resulting vulnerabilities are evident throughout development, and intervention before the challenges of increased independence during adolescence and adulthood may be especially important. There is a paucity of research and currently a lack of clear evidence-base for social skills training and advances in evidence-based intervention are especially important (but see Fisher et al., 2013; Thurman & Fisher, 2015). One of the struggles of intervention development, from feasibility studies to more thorough randomized controlled trials, is the rarity of this developmental disorder. Indeed, small sample sizes are a further hindrance to research endeavors and research groups across the world need to work toward "big data" and through collaboration we can build a far stronger evidence base concerning social behaviors, social vulnerabilities, and potential intervention strategies, while remaining vigilant of cultural variability.

APPENDIX

Interview Schedule: Adult Williams Syndrome Semistructured Interview

Section One: Social Profile

Remember, you don't have to answer any questions that you don't want to and you can stop the interview at any point, without giving a reason. We are going to start by talking about your friends, and what you like to do when you see them.

1. To begin with, can you tell me about the friends you had at school? (Prompts: how many close friends they had, how often they saw them, how they formed the friendships, what they did together, etc.)
2. Can you tell me about who your friends are now? (Prompts: how often they see them, what they do together)
3. When you meet someone for the first time (i.e., someone you don't know), what do you do?

   We are now going to talk about secrets.
4. Do you think you are good at keeping secrets? (Prompts: can you give me an example?)
5. Can you think of a time when it would not be OK to keep a secret?
6. Can you tell when someone else is lying to you or trying to trick you? (Prompts: can you give me an example?)
7. How do you know if you can trust someone?

Section Two: Computer Use

Now, we are going to talk about using the Internet.

8. How often do you go on the Internet?
9. Why do you go on the Internet? (Prompts: work, watch videos, go on Facebook.)

10. What is your favorite Website and why?
11. What do you think the best thing about having the Internet is?
12. What do you think the worst thing about the Internet is?
13. Do you use websites where you can talk to other people, such as Facebook?

If yes....

14. Who do you talk to on <insert name of Website>? (Prompts: how do you know them, have you met in real life, do you talk to people you have only met on the Internet?)
15. Has anything bad ever happened to you on the Internet? Can you tell me about it?
16. Do you think that your mum/dad worries about you when you're on the Internet?
17. Finally, do your parents set any rules for you when you're on the Internet? Do you follow these rules?

Thank you for answering these questions. If you want to ask any questions about the study, then I can answer them for you.

End of Interview

Interview Schedule: Parent Semi Structured Interview

Section One: General Profile

You are reminded that you do not have to answer any questions which you do not wish to. You can stop the interview at any point, without giving a reason. We are going to start with some general information on ______ and day-to-day living.

1. Can you please start by telling me a bit about ______, for example, their age, their daily routine, their interests...?
2. What would you say are the main challenges ______ faces on a day-to-day basis?
3. How, if at all, have these challenges changed as your son/daughter has grown up?
4. Can you tell me about any particular strength that ______ has and how s/he uses them? (for example, social, behavioral, hobby)
5. How does ______ fit into the structure of your immediate family, for example, do they have siblings? (if necessary probe the general family structure in terms of immediate family, involvement of grandparents, ages where relevant)

6. Does ______ have any other diagnoses? (for example, of another learning difficulty or developmental disorder and/or of any mental health difficulties?)

Section Two: Social Profile

I would now like to move on to talk about ______'s general social functioning. For this study we are especially interested in looking at social abilities. In this interview we are going to be thinking about ______'s abilities to interact with others, and to form and maintain relationships.

7. To begin, can you tell me about your son/daughter's peer social group during their school years? (for example, how many close friends they had, how often they saw them, how they formed the friendships, what they did together, etc.)
8. Can you now tell me about your son/daughter's current peer social group? What would you say the differences were between their peer social group now, compared to when _____ was a teenager?
9. Tell me a little bit more about their interaction style with people who are familiar to him/her? Has there been any change as they have grown up?
10. Can you also tell me about _____'s interaction style with people who are unfamiliar to him/her? Has there been any change as they have grown up?
11. Can you talk me through how ______ would interact with an unfamiliar person they had just met for the first time? We are going to go on to talk about some aspects of emotion and social behaviors, for example, _____'s trust behavior and awareness of deception.
12. Thinking about deception, can you tell me about ________'s ability to deceive others? Can you give me an example?
13. Can you also tell me about ________'s ability to recognize when someone else is lying? Can you give me an example?
14. How easy does _______ find it to trust other people? Can you give an example?

    What makes them more/less likely to trust someone?

    Do they ever change their mind about how trustworthy someone is?
15. Is there anything else that you feel is particularly important about the way in which _______ interacts with other people, for example, whether they suffer from anxiety?

Section Three: Computer Use

Technology is becoming an integral aspect of the lives of young people, offering new ways to play, socialize, and gain knowledge. For this section, I would like you to think about your son/daughter's computer usage, and in particular their use of the Internet.

16. Can you tell me about your son/daughter's computer usage, for example, how often they use it?
 Why do they use it?
 Do they use the Internet?
 What are their favorite Websites?

17. What do you worry about, if anything, when ______ is on the internet? Why does this make you worry?

18. Does _____ know that you're worried about this?

19. How aware is ______ of the potential dangers of the Internet? (ask about cyber-bullying, online grooming, inappropriate content, identity fraud.)

20. How aware would you say you are of these risks?

21. Do you take any precautions or set any rules for ________'s Internet use? If so, can you tell me about them and why you have set them?

22. Can you tell me about how easy or difficult you find it to monitor your son/daughter's Internet use? Can you tell me why?

23. What do you think the benefits are of ______ using the Internet? Can you give me some examples of how they have benefitted from having access to the Internet?

24. Is there anything else that you feel is particularly important about ______'s computer and Internet use that we have not already discussed?

Section Four: Risk and Resilience

Now that we have discussed _______'s offline and online world, we want you to think about their risk and resilience in these two environments. We will start by talking about the offline environment.

25. Can you tell me about how resilient you think ______ is? Can you tell me about a time when they coped well in a risky situation?

26. How vulnerable would you say your son/daughter is now? By vulnerable, we mean how "at risk" would you say your son/daughter is currently? How vulnerable were they when they were younger?

27. Is there anything that you can pinpoint that contributes to this vulnerability?

28. Can you give me an example of a time when they showed this vulnerability?
29. Can you give me an example of a time when they showed good resilience?
30. What strategies, if any, have you tried to promote resilience and reduce vulnerability? Were they effective?

Now we are going to talk about risk and resilience in the online environment, i.e., while _____ is on the Internet.

31. Can you tell me how resilient ______ is online? For example, how does s/he cope with upsetting information, how aware is s/he of potential dangers, does s/he know what to do if they are unhappy with anything that is said online?
32. Would you say the vulnerability experienced offline is the same or different to the vulnerability _______ faced online? What are the similarities? How are these environments different for _____?
33. What advice would you give to parents who are concerned about how vulnerable or at risk their son/daughter might be offline? Would this advice be the same if the vulnerability was online?
34. Finally, is there anything else you would like to add that you feel we haven't already covered?

Thank you for taking the time to participate in this research. If you have any questions for me I can try to answer them for you.

End of Interview

REFERENCES

Achenbach, T. M. (1991). *Manual for child behavior checklist/4-18 and 1991 profile*. Burlington, VT: University of Vermont, Dept. of Psychiatry.

Adolphs, R., Tranel, D., & Damasio, A. R. (1998). The human amygdala in social judgment. *Nature Reviews Genetics, 393*, 470–474.

Annaz, D., Karmiloff-Smith, A., Johnson, M. H., & Thomas, M. S. (2009). A cross-syndrome study of the development of holistic face recognition in children with autism, Down syndrome, and Williams syndrome. *Journal of experimental child psychology, 102*(4), 456–486.

Bellugi, U., Adolphs, R., Cassady, C., & Chiles, M. (1999). Towards the neural basis for hypersociability in a genetic syndrome. *Neuroreport, 10*(8), 1653–1657.

Bellugi, U., Wang, P. P., & Jernigan, T. L. (1994). Williams syndrome: An unusual neuropsychological profile. In S. Broman, & J. Grafman (Eds.), *Atypical cognitive deficits in developmental disorders: Implications for brain function* (pp. 23–56). Hillsdale: NJ: Erlbaum.

Braun, V., & Clarke, V. (2006). Using thematic analysis in psychology. *Qualitative Research in Psychology, 3*, 77–101.

Constantinno, J., & Gruber, C. (2005). *The social responsiveness scale*. Los Angeles, CA: Western Psychological Services.

Davies, M., Udwin, O., & Howlin, P. (1998). Adults with Williams syndrome. Preliminary study of social, emotional and behavioural difficulties. *The British Journal of Psychiatry, 172*, 273–276. http://dx.doi.org/10.1192/bjp.172.3.273.

Deruelle, C., Mancini, J., Livet, M. O., Casse-Perrot, C., & de Schonen, S. (1999). Configural and local processing of faces in children with Williams syndrome. *Brain and Cognition, 41*, 276–298.

Doyle, T. F., Bellugi, U., Korenberg, J. R., & Graham, J. (2004). "Everybody in the world is my friend" hypersociability in young children with Williams syndrome. *American Journal of Medical Genetics Part A, 124A*, 263–273.

D'Souza, D., & Karmiloff-Smith, A. (2011). When modularization fails to occur: A developmental perspective. *Cognitive Neuropsychology, 28*, 276–287.

Dykens, E. M. (2000). Psychopathology in children with intellectual disability. *Journal of Child Psychology and Psychiatry, 41*, 407–417.

Fidler, D. J., Hepburn, S. L., Most, D. E., Philofsky, A., & Rogers, S. J. (2007). Emotional responsivity in young children with Williams syndrome. *American Journal on Mental Retardation, 112*, 194–206.

Fisher, M. (2014). Evaluation of a stranger safety training programme for adults with Williams syndrome. *Journal of Intellectual Disability Research, 58*, 903–914. http://dx.doi.org/10.1111/jir.12108.

Fisher, M. H., Moskowitz, A., & Hodapp, R. M. (2013). Differences in social vulnerability among individuals with autism spectrum disorder, Williams syndrome, and Down syndrome. *Research in Autism Spectrum Disorders, 7*, 931–937. http://dx.doi.org/10.1016/j.rasd.2013.04.009.

van der Fluit, F., Gaffrey, M. S., & Klein-Tasman, B. P. (2012). Social cognition in Williams syndrome: Relations between performance on the social attribution task and cognitive and behavioral characteristics. *Frontiers in Developmental Psychology, 3*, 197.

Freeman, K., Williams, I. T., Farran, E., & Brown, J. (2010). Williams Syndrome: The extent of agreement between parent and self report of psychological difficulties. *European Journal of Psychiatry, 24*, 167–175.

Frigerio, E., Burt, D. M., Gagliardi, C., Cioffi, G., Martelli, S., Perrett, D. I., & Borgatti, R. (2006). Is everybody always my friend? Perception of approachability in Williams syndrome. *Neuropsychologia, 44*(2), 254–259.

Goldsmith, H. H., & Rothbart, M. K. (1991). Contemporary instruments for assessing early temperament by questionnaire and in the laboratory. In *Explorations in temperament* (pp. 249–272). US: Springer.

Grundy, E. (2006). Ageing and vulnerable elderly people: European perspectives. *Aging and Society, 26*(1), 105–134.

Hanley, M., Riby, D. M., Caswell, S., Rooney, S., & Back, E. (2013). Looking and thinking: How individuals with Williams syndrome make judgements about mental states. *Research in Developmental Disabilities, 34*, 4466–4476.

Hoffman, J. E., Landau, B., & Pagani, B. (2003). Spatial breakdown in spatial construction: Evidence from eye fixations in children with Williams syndrome. *Cognitive Psychology, 46*, 260–301.

Järvinen, A., & Bellugi, U. (2013). What does Williams syndrome reveal about the determinants of social behaviour? *Frontiers in Human Neuroscience, 7*, 321.

Järvinen, A., Korenberg, J. R., & Bellugi, U. (2013). The social phenotype of Williams syndrome. *Current Opinion in Neurobiology, 23*, 1–9. http://dx.doi.org/10.1016/j.conb.2012.12.006.

Jawaid, A., Riby, D. M., Owens, J., White, S. W., Tarar, T., & Schulz, P. E. (2012). 'Too withdrawn' or 'too friendly': Considering social vulnerability in two neurodevelopmental disorders. *Journal of Intellectual Disability Research, 56*, 335–350.

Jones, W., Bellugi, U., Lai, Z., Chiles, M., Reilly, J., Lincoln, A., & Adolphs, R. (2000). Hypersociability in Williams syndrome. *Journal of Cognitive Neuroscience, 12*(Suppl. 1), 30–46. http://dx.doi.org/10.1162/089892900561968.

Karmiloff-Smith, A., Brown, J. H., Grice, S., & Paterson, S. (2003). Dethroning the myth: Cognitive dissociations and innate modularity in Williams syndrome. *Developmental Neuropsychology, 23*, 229–244.

Karmiloff-Smith, A., Klima, E., Bellugi, U., Grant, J., & Baron-Cohen, S. (1995). Is there a social module? Language, face processing, and theory of mind in individuals with Williams Syndrome. *Journal of Cognitive Neuroscience*, 7(2), 196–208.

Karmiloff-Smith, A., Thomas, M., Annaz, D., Humphreys, K., Ewing, S., Brace, N., & Campbell, R. (2004). Exploring the Williams syndrome face-processing debate: The importance of building developmental trajectories. *Journal of Child Psychology and Psychiatry, 45*(7), 1258–1274.

Kennedy, D. P., Glascher, J., Tyszka, J., & Adolphs, R. (2009). Personal space regulation by the human amygdala. *Nature Neuroscience, 12*, 1226–1227.

Klein-Tasman, B. P., Li-Barber, K. T., & Magargee, E. T. (2011). Honing in on the social phenotype in Williams syndrome using multiple measures and multiple raters. *Journal of Autism and Developmental Disabilities, 41*, 341–351.

Levy, Y., & Herman, S. (2003). Morphological abilities of Hebrew-speaking adolescents with Williams syndrome. *Developmental Neuropsychology, 23*, 59–83.

Little, K., Riby, D. M., Janes, E., Clark, F., Fleck, R., & Rodgers, J. (2013). Heterogeneity of social approach behaviour in Williams syndrome: The role of response inhibition. *Research in Developmental Disabilities, 34*, 959–967.

Lough, E., & Fisher, M. (2016). Internet use and online safety in adults with Williams syndrome. *Journal of Intellectual Disability Research, 60*, 1020–1030.

Lough, E., Flynn, E., & Riby, D. M. (2015). Mapping real-world to online vulnerability in young people with developmental disorders: Illustrations from autism and Williams syndrome. *Review Journal of Autism and Developmental Disorders, 2*, 1–7. http://dx.doi.org/10.1007/s40489-014-0029-2.

Lough, E., Flynn, E., & Riby, D. M. (2016). Personal space regulation in Williams syndrome: The effect of familiarity. *Journal of Autism and Developmental Disorders, 10*, 3207–3215.

Lough, E., Hanley, M., Rodgers, J., South, M., Kirk, H., Kennedy, D. P., & Riby, D. M. (2015). Violations of personal space in young people with autism spectrum disorders and Williams syndrome: Insights from the Social Responsiveness Scale. *Journal of Autism and Developmental Disorders, 45*(12), 4101–4108.

Lough, E., Rodgers, J., Janes, E., Little, K., & Riby, D. M. (2016). Parent insights into atypicalities of social approach behaviour in Williams syndrome. *Journal of Intellectual Disability Research., 60*, 1097–1108.

Martens, M. A., Hasinski, A. E., Andridge, R. R., & Cunningham, W. A. (2012). Continuous cognitive dynamics of the evaluation of trustworthiness in Williams syndrome. *Frontiers in psychology, 3*, 160.

Ng, R., Fillet, P., DeWitt, M., Heyman, G. D., & Bellugi, U. (2015). Reasoning about trust among individuals with Williams syndrome. *American Journal on Intellectual and Developmental disabilities, 12*, 527–541.

Plesa-Skwerer, D., Faja, S., Schofield, C., Verbalis, A., & Tager-Flusberg, H. (2006). Perceiving facial and vocal expressions of emotion in individuals with Williams syndrome. *American Journal on Mental Retardation, 111*(1), 15–26.

Porter, M. A., Coltheart, M., & Langdon, R. (2007). The neuropsychological basis of hypersociability in Williams and Down syndrome. *Neuropsychologia, 45*(12), 2839–2849.

Riby, D. M., & Hancock, P. J. B. (2008). Viewing it differently: Social scene perception in Williams syndrome and autism. *Neuropsychologia, 46*, 2855–2860.
Riby, D. M., Hanley, M., Kirk, H., Clark, F., Little, K., Fleck, R., … Rodgers, J. (2014). The interplay between anxiety and social functioning in Williams syndrome. *Journal of Autism and Developmental Disorders, 44*, 1220–1229.
Riby, D. M., Kirk, H., Hanley, M., & Riby, L. M. (2014). Stranger danger awareness in Williams syndrome. *Journal of Intellectual Disability Research, 58*, 572–582. http://dx.doi.org/10.1111/jir.12055.
Rosner, B. A., Hodapp, R. M., Fidler, D. J., Sagun, J. N., & Dykens, E. M. (2004). Social competence in persons with Prader-Willi, Williams and Down's syndromes. *Journal of Applied Research in Intellectual Disabilities, 17*(3), 209–217.
Searcy, Y. M., Lincoln, A. J., Rose, F. E., Klima, E. S., Bavar, N., & Korenberg, J. R. (2004). The relationship between age and IQ in adults with Williams syndrome. *American Journal on Mental Retardation, 109*, 231–236.
Thurman, A. E., & Fisher, M. H. (2015). The Williams syndrome social phenotype: Disentangling the contributions of social interest and social difficulties. *International Review of Research in Developmental Disabilities, 49*, 191–227.
Udwin, O. (1990). A survey of adults with Williams syndrome and idiopathic infantile hypercalcaemia. *Developmental Medicine and Child Neurology, 32*, 129–141.
Viera, A. J., & Garrett, J. M. (2005). Understanding inter-observer agreement: The kappa statistic. *Family Medicine, 37*(5), 360–363.
Wells, M., & Mitchell, K. J. (2013). Patterns of Internet use and risk of online victimization for youth with and without disabilities. *Journal of Special Education, 20*, 1–10.

CHAPTER SEVEN

Sexual Health of People With an Intellectual Disability

Joke M.T. Stoffelen[*,§,||,1], **Dilana Schaafsma**[*,¶,||], **Gerjo Kok**[*,||], **Leopold M.G. Curfs**[*,||]
[*]Maastricht University, Maastricht, The Netherlands
[§]Zorgbelang Gelderland-Utrecht, Arnhem, The Netherlands
[¶]Fontys University of Applied Sciences, Eindhoven, The Netherlands
[||]The Governor Kremers Centre, Maastricht, The Netherlands
[1]Corresponding author: E-mail: joke.stoffelen@maastrichtuniversity.nl

Contents

International Review of Research in Developmental Disabilities, Volume 52
ISSN 2211-6095
http://dx.doi.org/10.1016/bs.irrdd.2017.07.004

Abstract

People have sexual needs, expressions, drives, and desires. Sexuality should be a positive part of the human experience and human life. People with an intellectual disability, like everyone else, have sexual feelings, needs, and desires. However, some aspects can be essentially different for them. This warrants special attention.

1. INTRODUCTION

All people have sexual needs, expressions, drives, and desires. According to Aristoteles (the Greek philosopher who lived in ancient times), we are "social animals, not made to live alone." In essence, people want to contact other human beings for friendship, support, recognition, acceptance, and sex. These forms of contact empower people "to live more effectively, more healthily, and for longer" (Pahl, 2000, p. 149).

Nussbaum (2014, p. 57) describes sexuality as an essential human capability: "Having the opportunity for sexual satisfaction and choices about reproduction." Further, the World Association for Sexual Health (WAS) promotes sexual health by developing sexual rights for all. The WAS (2014) has specified a number of sexual health rights, including the right to privacy, the right to sexual health, the right to marriage and to start a family, the right to decide on the number of children, the right to information and education, the right to freedom of opinion and expression, and the right to protection of these rights. Unfortunately, many different religious traditions have created different laws, doctrines, and traditions regarding (un)acceptable sexual behaviors (Westheimer, 2005) that might not be in concordance with these rights.

Sexuality should be a positive part of the human experience and human life. As such, these rights are afforded to all people, including those with a disability. People with an intellectual disability (ID), like everyone else, have sexual feelings, needs, and desires. However, some aspects can be fundamentally different for them. These differences warrant special attention.

According to recent estimates, 1.04% of the global population has an ID (Maulik, Mascarenhas, Mathers, Dua, & Saxena, 2011). Just as the population of people with an ID is very diverse (Chiurazzi & Pirozzi, 2016), so too are they diverse in terms of sexual experiences, sexual desires and needs, and sexual knowledge (Schaafsma, Kok, Stoffelen, & Curfs, 2017). Sexuality surrounds us every day and we encounter "concerns," "issues," and "questions." People with ID also have specific problems with sexuality and their own concerns, issues, and questions.

The objective of this chapter is to provide an overview of issues concerning sexuality and gender in people with an ID. We describe what can be different for them and why, and what the important items are concerning sexuality. To begin, we focus briefly on the concept of ID and on the heterogeneity of the group of people with an ID. We explain various syndromes that are linked with ID and their experiences with sexuality and gender. In the third section, we address the sexual rights of people with an ID and how sexual rights are a starting point and an important basis for providing high-quality care and support. In Section 4 we discuss a number of focus points, including people with severe and profound IDs, relationships, identifying sexual abuse, and enjoyable, safe sex, and sexual empowerment. In Section 5 we address the gender differences in people with an ID in relation to sexuality, and in Section 6 we focus on sexual diversity, a rather neglected topic for people with ID. In Section 7 we discuss the research that has been conducted in the Netherlands to provide support to people with ID who have experienced sexual problems and who identify as homosexual. Finally, Section 8 contains some concluding remarks.

2. CHARACTERISTICS OF INTELLECTUAL DISABILITY

ID, as defined by the Diagnostic and Statistical Manual of Mental Disorders, Fifth Edition (DSM-5; American Psychiatric Association, 2013), is characterized by a substantial impairment in both cognitive functioning (an IQ of below 70) and adaptive behavior, originating in the developmental period (before age 18). Impairments can impact a range of skills, including conceptual skills (such as reading and writing, understanding money, time, and numbers), social skills (such as interpersonal relationships, self-confidence, obeying rules and laws, avoiding victimization), and practical adaptive skills (including activities of daily living, dealing with money, health care, and safety).

The definitions of ID are not unequivocal. The conceptual framework is also subject to change (Schalock et al., 2010, 2012). For a description of the concept of ID and an explanation of the context of the definitions used, see de Bruijn, Buntinx, and Twint (2014).

Traditionally, intellectual functioning is subdivided into various levels (World Health Organization, 2016), including

- Mild ID: IQ 50/55-70;
- Moderate ID: IQ 35/40-50/55;
- Severe ID: IQ 20/25-35/40;
- Profound ID: IQ below 20/25.

2.1 Specific Syndromes, Sexuality, and Gender

Genetic factors can increase the risk of ID (Veltman & Brunner, 2012) and play an important role in the development of developmental disorders. This often occurs not only among those with severe or profound ID but also to people with mild ID (de Ligt et al., 2012). Just as individuals with different genetic syndromes display distinct behavior profiles (Dykens & Hodapp, 1999), individuals with various genetic syndromes (e.g., Prader—Willi syndrome or Down syndrome) may differentially experience aberrant sexual development or sexual health. In many genetic syndromes, the sexual development or sexual health is so aberrant and sometimes gender-specific that it can have consequences for providing effective care and support to people with both an ID and a specific syndrome. Here, we describe the five most well-known syndromes in people with ID in relation to sexuality: Down syndrome, Prader—Willi syndrome, Williams syndrome, Fragile X syndrome, and Fetal Alcohol syndrome (FAS). Table 1 provides an overview

Table 1 Overview of Specific Syndromes and Corresponding Issues Concerning Sexuality and Gender

Syndrome	Characteristics
Down syndrome	• Pubertal development is often incomplete • Males are often infertile • Males have a higher risk of testicular cancer • Females have a lower risk of breast cancer • In females menopause begins earlier
Prader—Willi syndrome (PWS)	• Reduced levels of sex hormones in boys after the age of 9: No deepening of the voice, little male hair growth (however, pubic hair appears earlier than in their peers) • In girls: Breast development is indistinguishable from fat accumulation, menstruation is rare, menstrual cycle disturbances occur after puberty, and fertility is reduced • People with PWS also have sexual feelings and sexual needs. Sex education should be provided, with a focus on preventing sexual abuse

Table 1 Overview of Specific Syndromes and Corresponding Issues Concerning Sexuality and Gender—cont'd

Syndrome	Characteristics
Williams syndrome	• Early onset of puberty; growth spurt in puberty • Vulnerability to sexual abuse due to the tendency to be overly friendly with strangers, a lack of social judgment skills, and a limited social network • Inability to deal effectively with menstruation • Early menopause
Fragile X syndrome	• Boys have large testes • Girls experience early puberty and premenstrual syndrome
Cornelia de Lange syndrome	• Boys have a high likelihood of undescended testes • Growth spurt in puberty
Smith–Magenis syndrome	• Carriers of a specific mutation may have polyembolokoilamania (the tendency to insert objects into body openings) • Early onset of puberty • Premature menopause • Children tend to engage in "self-hugging" when excited • In girls there is a relationship between increased behavioral problems and the menstrual cycle
Congenital infections: Rubella, herpes infection, toxoplasmosis	• Sexual development can be disrupted • Menstrual problems: Irregular menstruation and premenstrual syndrome • Early menopause
Klinefelter syndrome	Occurs only in boys • Small penis and small testes, breast growth, reduced muscle mass, and feminine distribution of body fat • Delayed or incomplete puberty: little body hair • In males: Decreased libido, reduced muscle mass and reduced bone mass, infertility (99%–100%), increased risk of breast cancer
Turner syndrome	Occurs only in girls • No breast development • Spontaneous puberty, but late stagnation occurs in 10%–20% • Infertility (95%–98%)
Sotos syndrome	• Early onset of puberty; • In girls: Irregular menstruation • Emotional vulnerability and low self-confidence
Neurofibromatosis	• During puberty: delayed growth or excessively rapid development • Women under the age of 50 have a 50-fold increased risk of breast cancer

(Continued)

Table 1 Overview of Specific Syndromes and Corresponding Issues Concerning Sexuality and Gender—cont'd

Syndrome	Characteristics
Charge syndrome	• Delayed or absent puberty, resulting in aberrant growth • In boys: low testosterone levels • In girls: Ovulation dysfunction
Fetal Alcohol syndrome	Prone to sexually deviant behavior
Rubinstein–Taybi syndrome	• In boys: incomplete or delayed descent of testes (78%–100%) • Genital abnormalities: Hypospadias in 11% of the boys: the urethra is too short and the urinary opening is not at the head of the penis; occasionally a minor to severe downward bending of the penis when erect; • In girls: Heavy menstruation and metrorrhagia (bleeding from the uterus outside the menstrual period)
1p36 Deletion syndrome	• Puberty can begin earlier or later than normal • Genital abnormalities: Hypospadias in boys and hypoplasia (incomplete development) in boys and girls
Congenital defects in glycosylation	• In girls: Absence of puberty; no pregnancies are known • In boys: normal puberty, testes are often shrunken
Wolf–Hirschhorn syndrome	• All people known to have this syndrome have been infertile • Genital abnormalities: in boys hypospadias and cryptorchidism (undescended testes); in girls aplasia/hypoplasia of the clitoris (excessive or inadequate development), congenital abnormalities of the uterus or vagina, and streak gonads (empty fibrous tissue instead of gonads)
Phelan–McDermid or 22q13.3 Deletion syndrome	• Pubertal development and menstruation proceed normally • Nothing is known about fertility
Lesch–Nyhan syndrome	• Puberty is often delayed • Testes are sometimes underdeveloped

of 19 additional syndromes, with related characteristics concerning some aspect of sexuality. Please note, not all of the syndromes are always genetic (e.g., FAS) or linked with ID (e.g., Turner syndrome and Klinefelter syndrome). Further, the descriptions only provide an image of people with a particular syndrome. In several syndromes, the behavioral phenotypes can change with age. And furthermore there can be a within-group variation (Hodapp & Dykens, 2004).

2.2 Down Syndrome

Down syndrome occurs when an individual has a full or partial extra copy of chromosome 21. A few of the common physical traits of Down syndrome are low muscle tone, small stature, an upward slant to the eyes, and a single deep crease across the center of the palm. Each person with Down syndrome is a unique individual and may possess these characteristics to different degrees, or not at all (Rex & Preus, 1982; Kraijer & Plas, 2007). There are several characteristics concerning sexuality related to individuals with Down syndrome. First, the pubertal development is often incomplete in people with Down syndrome. Second, males are often infertile and have a higher risk of testicular cancer. Finally, females have a lower risk of breast cancer and menopause begins earlier (Beumer & Bevers, 2014).

2.3 Prader—Willi Syndrome

Prader—Willi syndrome is the most common known genetic cause of life-threatening obesity in children. Although the cause is complex, it results from an abnormality on the 15th chromosome. It occurs in males and females equally and in all races (Holm et al., 1993; Kraijer & Plas, 2007). There are several characteristics concerning sexuality for individuals with Prader—Willi syndrome. First, there is a difference in sexual development between boys and girls. Specifically, there is a reduced level of sex hormones in boys after the age of 9, resulting in no deepening of the voice and little male hair growth (however, pubic hair appears earlier than in their peers). In girls, the breast development is indistinguishable from fat accumulation, menstruation is rare, menstrual cycle disturbances occur after puberty, and fertility is reduced (Hendrikx & Mulder, 2016).

2.4 Williams Syndrome

Williams syndrome is a genetic condition that is present at birth and can affect males and females and all races equally. It is characterized by medical problems, including cardiovascular disease, developmental delays, and learning challenges. These often occur side by side with striking verbal abilities, highly social personalities, and an affinity for music (Kraijer & Plas, 2007). In regard to sexuality (Bankras, van Loon, & Reijenga, 2011), young people with Williams syndrome have an early onset of puberty and a growth spurt. Because of their tendency to be overly friendly with strangers, their lack of social judgment skills, and a limited social network, individuals with Williams syndrome are vulnerable to sexual abuse. Young girls and women are often unable to deal effectively with menstruation and experience an early menopause (Bankras et al., 2011).

2.5 Fragile X Syndrome

Persons with Fragile X syndrome often have ID (most mild to moderate). Usually, males are more severely affected by this disorder than females. One-third of individuals with Fragile X syndrome also have an autism spectrum disorder. There may be an elongated head, big ears, a high forehead, a big chin, dental crowding, hyperlaxity, flat feet, and often a soft velvety skin (Kraijer & Plas, 2007). Characteristics concerning sexuality include boys with Fragile X syndrome have large testes and girls experience early puberty and premenstrual syndrome (Peters & Safi, 2012).

2.6 Fetal Alcohol Syndrome

Fetal Alcohol Spectrum Disorder (FAS and FASD) is a set of congenital abnormalities due to alcohol use in pregnancy. Effects of alcohol on the child consist of physical, mental, behavioral, and/or learning problems that have consequences throughout life. Individuals with FAS or FASD are prone to sexually deviant behavior (Demirdas, Ganzevoort, & Fischer, 2016). In their research, Streissguth et al. (2004) reported inappropriate sexual behavior, such as making inappropriate sexual advances or inappropriate sexual touching, compulsive sexual behavior, and masturbating in public.

3. SEXUAL RIGHTS

People with ID have human rights (Stainton & Clare, 2012), including sexual rights. According to the American Association on Intellectual and Developmental Disabilities (AAIDD), "These sexual rights and needs must be affirmed, defended, and respected" (in "Position Statement Sexuality" AAIDD, 2008). The World Health Organization (2015) also cited specific rights for people with ID: they have the right to sexual and reproductive health services, the right to decide about their own fertility, the right to information and education about sexual health, and people with a disability must not be compelled to undergo involuntary procedures such as sterilization.

3.1 Rights Cannot Be Taken for Granted

Having sexual rights and exercising these rights in daily life cannot be taken for granted by people with an ID (Ignagni, Fudge Schormans, Liddiard, & Runswick-Cole, 2016; Watson, Venema, Molloy, & Reich, 2002). Unfortunately, many individuals with ID are not given the respect and support that is required to realize these sexual rights. Watson et al. (2002) indicate examples as "a lack of privacy, inability to find a partner, and restrictive institutional policies or rules" as barrier to exercising their sexual rights. For people with an ID who live in an institution, the right to privacy is poorly acknowledged (Hollomotz, 2008). Further, because of overprotection, segregation, and a lack of social skills, people with an ID are especially vulnerable to sexual abuse (Hollomotz, 2011). Hollomotz (2011) interviewed 29 people with a mild ID (12 men and 17 women) to explore the social causes for the risk of sexual violence and reported,

> *...He brought a games console, cause he knew I likes games and he brought a games console in to specifically...I think the phrase 'give me a hand' while I was playing on the games console...I won't go down how it escalated from that. It did...and then you elbow them in the face to get them off you and they go and tell on you because they raped you. They say you raped them.*
>
> ***Hollomotz (2011, p. 71)***

3.2 The Right to Protection

Sexual abuse has been a serious problem for people with ID for many years. The figures for sexual abuse range, indicating that from 25% to 82% of individuals with intellectual and developmental disabilities (IDD) experience sexual abuse (Abbott & Howarth, 2005; Eastgate, Van Driel, Lennox, & Scheermeyer, 2011; Hickson, Khemka, Golden, & Chatzistyli, 2008; McCarthy, 2001; Reiter, Bryen, & Shachar, 2007; Stoffelen, Kok, Hospers, & Curfs, 2013; Van Berlo et al., 2011). Others have reported that the risk of sexual abuse for people with an ID is estimated to be three times higher than for people without ID (Rapport commissie Samson, 2012; Reiter et al., 2007; Van Berlo et al., 2011). Even studies examining the sexuality of people with an ID, not specifically focusing on abuse, have reported incidents of sexual abuse in this group (Schaafsma, Stoffelen, Kok, & Curfs, 2013; Stoffelen et al., 2013). Reiter et al. (2007) found that young people with an ID are more often abused than young people without a disability, and they are more likely to be forced to do things they do not want to do.

Approximately 40% of the respondents with ID in their study had been subjected to sexual abuse (Reiter et al., 2007).

People with an ID are especially vulnerable to sexual abuse, in part, because of a lack of knowledge (Fyson & Kitson, 2010). People with an ID receive less education about sexuality. As a result, they usually have less knowledge about topics such as masturbation, pregnancy, safe sex, reproduction, and sexual diversity than their peers without an ID (Healy et al., 2009; Kelly, Crowley, & Hamilton, 2009; Lesseliers, 1999; Leutar & Mihoković, 2007; McCabe, 1999; McCarthy, 2009; Murphy & O'Callaghan, 2004; Schaafsma et al., 2017). In one study by McCarthy (2009), 14 out of 23 women did not know how their conception worked, 11 lacked knowledge about reproduction, 6 were not familiar with menopause, and 1 did not understand the connection between sex and pregnancy. McCarthy (2014) further reported one women's passivity regarding taking contraception "I don't ask, I just go and have it (contraception), I don't ask."

Moreover, social skills, communication skills, and decision-making skills are often inadequate for individuals with ID (Egemo-Helm et al., 2007; Hayashi, Arakida, & Ohashi, 2011; Khemka, Hickson, & Reynolds, 2005; McCarthy, 2014; Miltenberger et al., 1999). Lack of knowledge and skills concerning sexuality can result in someone being less capable of recognizing risky situations, which in turn increases the risk of sexual abuse (Schaafsma, 2013). Another important factor is the dependence on others for care and support. In their daily lives, individuals with ID come into contact with many professional carers (Löfgren-Mårtenson, 2004; Stoffelen, Schaafsma, Kok, & Curfs, 2017). This support relationship is characterized not only by dependence but also by a difference in power. This kind of support relationship makes a person with an ID even more vulnerable, especially if someone in his or her environment has malicious intentions. The dependency is related to a lack of empowerment. For many people with an ID, it is difficult to take action if they experience something unpleasant, which is partly because they are not always taken seriously but also because they do not know how they should act in such situations (Scharlo, Ebbers, & Spijker, 2014, p. 19).

Finally, sexual abuse has a major impact on the lives of victims. Experiences with sexual abuse can lead to severe mental problems such as depression and anxiety (Sequeira, Howlin, & Hollins, 2003). Hickson et al. (2008) concluded that women with ID with a history of sexual abuse struggle more with decision-making than women with ID who had not been subjected to sexual abuse. They also experience more stress, have more comorbidity with other conditions, and more frequently need to receive therapeutic support. Sequeira et al. (2003) reported similar findings, as they found that individuals with ID who were victims of sexual abuse often have more psychiatric and behavioral problems.

3.3 The Right to Information and Education

A lack of knowledge about sexuality and sexual rights makes people with an ID especially vulnerable (Murphy & O'Callaghan, 2004; O'Callaghan & Murphy, 2007). In O'Callaghan and Murphy's (2007) study, approximately half of the participants thought they were not allowed to have sex. In their opinion, it was illegal. Alternatively, participants were unsure as to whether or not they were legally allowed to have sex. In the same study, half of the adults with an ID did not know that there are laws that protect them from having to engage in sexual activities with guardians or caretakers.

When it comes to exercising their sexual rights, people with ID encounter resistance in their immediate surroundings (Bernert, 2011; McGuire & Bayley, 2011). For example, family members and staff carers often have different standards for people with an ID than they do for themselves, and they are often resistant to allowing education about sexuality and sexual rights (Christian, Stinson, & Dotson, 2001; Evans, McGuire, Healy, & Carley, 2009; Swango-Wilson, 2008; Yool, Langdon, & Garner, 2003). A questionnaire among family (n = 155) and care staff (n = 153) indicated significant differences in opinions between family and care staff (Evans et al., 2009). Care staff was more likely to support people with ID in (sexual) relationships, whereas family carers accepted only platonic friendships and nonintimate relationships. Eighty percent of the family carers did not support sexual relationships of people with ID. Young, Gore, and McCarthy (2012) found in semistructured interviews with 10 staff members attitudes that correlate with negative, traditional, and gender stereotypes; men with an ID were perceived as sexually motivated and women with an ID as sexually innocent.

People with an ID also have little access to information about their rights due to the inaccessible language used in the human rights documents. Stories and personal biographies in understandable language can enable people with an ID to understand these rights and exercise them in their daily lives (Abbott, 2013). Training and support can help people with ID, family members, and carers talk about the sensitive topic of sexuality (Abbott & Howarth, 2005; Evans et al., 2009; Stoffelen et al., 2013). A study conducted among 39 participants with an ID showed that they are fully capable of indicating what they think is important: a respectful relationship, feeling safe, and being able to choose your living companions yourself (Stoffelen et al., 2017). Unfortunately, Evans et al. (2009) found low levels of staff training (12%) and low levels of family carer training regarding sexual education (8%), indicating a need for further training and support.

3.4 The Right to Have Children

Of all sexual rights, the right for individuals with ID to have children is one of the most controversial in society (Hendriks & Legemaate, 2009). In the Netherlands, a disincentive policy regarding sexual expressions for people with IDs is in force (VWS, 2004; 2006), despite the opposing views of the Health Council of the Netherlands, associations of parents of children with disabilities, the Royal Dutch Society for the Promotion of Medicine, and legal frameworks such as the European Convention on Human Rights and the Medical Treatment Agreement Act (Kalthoff, 2015).

Parents with an ID are a very heterogeneous group. There are parents with or without an institutional history and parents without the "label" of ID. Regardless, they all experience barriers while fulfilling their role as parents, such as social pressure not to have children or to have an abortion, and the fear and pressure that their children will be taken away from them after they are born. In addition, these parents often have to deal with stress, depression, and poor mental health, and they tend to have a smaller social network. In response to these pressures, a position paper from the International Association for the Scientific Study of Intellectual and Developmental Disabilities (IASSIDD) project group recommended that the label "ID" should not be directly equivalent to "incompetent" parenthood. Rather, they recommended giving more attention and support to vulnerable families (Llewellyn, Traustadóttir, McConnell, & Sigurjónsdóttir, 2010).

Children of parents with an ID do grow up in an environment with a multiplicity of problems: they are more likely to live in an unsafe situation, they are often stigmatized, and their parents often have financial problems (Kalthoff, 2015). Research shows, however, that parents with ID who have lower scores of social adaptability benefit from video training (Hodes, 2017). The Video-Feedback Intervention for Positive Parenting with the focus on Sensitive Discipline (VIPP-SD) showed parents videos of educational situations and reviewed them with the parents with ID. As a result, parents learned to see the child's perspective and they developed more empathy, which made them more sensitive to their child's needs.

Finally, Llewellyn et al. (2010) pointed out that the term "parents with an ID" usually concerns the mothers. In the scientific literature, and in research and in health care, little attention is paid to the fathers and their perspective. Llewellyn et al. (2010) advocate to include fathers and to compare parents with ID with parents without ID to gain more knowledge on how the ID of parents influences their parenting skills.

4. POINTS OF INTEREST

As stated previously, people with an ID experience a variety of problems in the area of sexuality. These problems are not only due to the characteristics of an ID but also due to environmental factors that may impact the individual with IDD. People with an ID often require support throughout their lives to function as normally as possible in society, and this need for support also extends to the area of sexuality.

4.1 People With Severe and Profound Intellectual Disability

In research into sexuality, virtually no attention is paid to people with a severe ID (Duke, 2011; Hubert, 2009; Kok, Maassen, Maaskant, & Curfs, 2009). In one of the only studies, Hubert (2009) used ethnographic methods for research with people with severe ID and found that individuals with severe ID are extremely dependent on others. They had no control over their sexual expression and intimate relationships. Further, their sexual experiences appeared to be primarily physical in nature. Kok et al. (2009) interviewed 12 staff members, all with more than five years of work experience with people with severe ID. Carers indicated that it is difficult to assess the sexual needs or preferences of people with severe ID due to their intellectual and communicative limitations and behavioral problems. Overall, individuals with severe and very severe IDs experience inadequate care and support in the area of sexuality (Kok et al., 2009).

I think that it would be good if we knew more about the sexuality of our clients. During my training, sexuality was discussed only theoretically and was not applied to clients. And all the courses that I have taken are about people with mild intellectual disabilities. We don't know nearly enough about the sexual development of our clients.

Female who works with people with severe ID, 8 years of experience, in Kok et al., (2009, p. 203).

4.2 Relationships

People with an ID report various problems regarding finding, entering into, and maintaining friendships and sexual relationships (Abbott & Burns, 2007; Abbott & Howarth, 2007). These problems are reflected, for example, in the size of their social networks; these are smaller relative to the networks of people without an ID (Hollomotz, 2011). Loneliness is also a major problem for people with an ID. There are indications that half of the individuals with an ID are lonely, while 15%—30% of the people without ID are lonely (Gilmore & Cuskelly, 2014). A theoretical model of vulnerability comprises three important domains: social attitudes and expectations; opportunities and experiences; and skills. Deficits or problems in these domains may result in loneliness. Gilmore and Cuskelly (2014) highlight the need to apply the model of vulnerability to understand the experiences of loneliness of people with ID.

A number of conditions contribute to problems with forming personal relationships, starting with the ID itself. As stated previously (de Bruijn et al., 2014; Gilmore & Cuskelly, 2014; Schalock et al., 2010, 2012; WHO, 2016), an ID is characterized by limitations in cognitive functioning and adaptive behavior, including limitations in social and communicative skills, which are essential to personal relationships.

The environment also contributes to problems with personal (and sexual) relationships (Gilmore & Cuskelly, 2014). People with an ID are often dependent on others (i.e., their parents or professional carers) for care and support. This dependence on others means that they are also dependent on them for information and sex education (Schaafsma, Kok, Stoffelen, van Doorn, & Curfs, 2014). Research has shown that people with an ID receive little or no education about sexuality (Levy & Packman, 2004; McCabe, Cummins, & Deeks, 1999; Murphy & O'Callaghan, 2004; Schaafsma, 2013; Schaafsma et al., 2013). Murphy and O'Callaghan (2004) assessed the sexual knowledge and vulnerability for sexual abuse among 60 young adults with ID and 60 young adults without ID. Adults with ID were significantly less well-informed on almost all aspects of sex. Further, if individuals with ID do receive sex education, then they often have difficulty remembering the information (Löfgren-Mårtenson, 2012).

Why are people with an ID given so little suitable education, despite all the problems surrounding sexuality and the obvious fact that they have difficulty understanding and remembering information? Despite the increasingly positive attitudes with respect to the sexuality of people with an ID (Christian et al., 2001; Cuskelly & Bryde, 2004; Lafferty, McConkey, & Simpson, 2012; Rohleder, Braathen, Swartz, & Eide, 2009), research indicates that sexuality is still seen as a taboo topic (Bernert & Ogletree, 2013; Löfgren-Mårtenson, 2004; McCabe et al., 1999; Rohleder, 2010). In others words, you should not talk about sex or sexuality with individuals with ID. This lack of talking about sexuality could explain why family members and professional carers do not address the topic of sexuality sufficiently (Abbott & Burns, 2007; Abbott & Howarth, 2007; Kok et al., 2009). For example, one individual with ID stated, "I tried to talk to my mum about it but she just blew up, and she said, If you go on and on about it, I'll take you out of the center" (female in Abbott & Burns, 2007).

As a result, individuals with ID often do not understand how they should deal with questions related to sexuality (Howard-Barr, Rienzo, Pigg, & James, 2005) and consequently act inappropriately (Evans et al., 2009). They are also sometimes given inconsistent information. For example, one carer could approve of someone being in a relationship, while another carer would disapprove of a relationship.

The perceptions and attitudes of individuals working with people with an ID have also played a role in their inability to have appropriate sexual relationships. After all, why would you provide sex education to someone if you do not acknowledge that they have sexual needs or you do not recognize those needs? Although many people with an ID indicate that they want to have sexual relationships, the environment discourages these kind of relationships (Healy, McGuire, Evans, & Carley, 2009; Kelly et al., 2009; Löfgren-Mårtenson, 2004). On the one hand, these reactions by care staff and family members are a result from fear of pregnancy or sexual abuse. On the other hand, it is due to the stigmatization of people with an ID being "eternal children" (Wilkinson, Theodore, & Raczka, 2015) and/or that they exist in a state of permanent adolescence (Hollomotz, 2011). Sexual activities are incompatible with these stigmatized images. In cases where sex education is provided in an organization, then, it is often in response to questions or problems, instead of proactive, preventative education (Abbott & Burns, 2007; Abbott & Howarth, 2007; Schaafsma et al., 2014).

Moreover, there is often no room for sexual experimentation. Löfgren-Mårtenson (2004, p. 205) notes a difference between male and female staff members:

> *...female staff members are more restrictive concerning sexual expression among the young adults. In contrast, their male counterparts tend to allow increased sexual expression and are more open to letting it 'go further' than the female staff members. Since so few men work in the field, the consequence is a female world with a restrictive set of rules. The female staff members focus primarily on the male's sexual behaviour in order to protect the young women.*

In short, many gains can still be made in the area of personal relationships. Enlarging the social networks of individuals with ID and improving their qualities is an important initial step. In addition, attention should also be paid to increasing the knowledge, skills, and attitudes of individuals working with individuals with ID concerning personal relationships. Professional carers and family members play an important role in this process (Abbott & Burns, 2007; Healy et al., 2009; Kelly et al., 2009; Löfgren-Mårtenson, 2004; Schaafsma et al., 2014).

4.3 Signs of Sexual Abuse

Often individuals with ID might not be aware that abuse has occurred or understand that sexual abuse has happened, making it important for others to know and recognize signs of abuse (Scharlo et al., 2014; Stoffelen et al., 2013). For example, sex could take place voluntarily, but involving an undesirable difference in power, such as between a client and his/her carer. For example, one individual stated, "It happened at night. Then they come to you. Then they wake you up" (male, aged 53, in Stoffelen et al., 2013, p. 260).

Sexual abuse can be detected in various ways (Heestermans, van den Boogaard, & Embregts, 2015). Of course, the clearest signal is when a third party sees the actual abuse taking place. Detection can also result from a disclosure—perhaps spontaneous—by the victim, when they tell someone else about the abuse, deliberately or otherwise.

Direct signals can also indicate abuse, such as a minor with a sexually transmittable disease or a mentally incompetent woman with a severe ID who is found to be pregnant. A vague (possibly spontaneous) disclosure can also be a sign of sexual abuse (Heestermans et al., 2015). For example, a client may report that he/she no longer wants to play with a neighbor because the activities are too painful.

Finally, indirect signals may also indicate abuse. These can not only be physical signals, such as mysterious wounds around the genitals and/or rectum, but also behavioral signals such as various types of pain, anxiety, or problem behavior. It is important to consider that the injuries may also have other causes that are unrelated to abuse and to conduct a full assessment before jumping to conclusions (Heestermans et al., 2015).

4.4 Sexual Empowerment

Although individual and environmental factors can increase the vulnerability to sexual abuse of someone with an ID, such factors can also reduce vulnerability. At the individual level, more attention should be paid to increasing skills, such as decision-making skills (Khemka et al., 2005) and knowledge related to empowerment. Professional carers and family members have an important responsibility in this regard (Heestermans et al., 2015). They could, for example, provide proper training to individuals with ID.

5. SEXUALITY AND GENDER

In very general terms, two types of sex can be distinguished: solo sex and sex with a partner. Safe sex is defined as having sex without the risk of sexually transmitted diseases (STDs) and unplanned pregnancy. Enjoyable or pleasurable sex is defined as having sexual experiences that are free of coercion and take place without pain or negative feelings. Unfortunately, positive sexual experiences are rare in people with IDs in comparison to their peers without ID (Leutar & Mihoković, 2007; McCabe, 1999; Siebelink, de Jong, Taal, & Roelvink, 2006). In part, this lack of positive feelings has to do with the above-mentioned aspects, such as lack of knowledge, skills, support, or the possibility to engage in experimentation. Moreover, the sexual experiences of males and females with an ID also differ. In this next section, we explore the differences between men and women with ID.

In the scientific literature on sexuality and people with an ID, a distinction is not always made regarding gender. Porter, Christian, and Poling (2003) screened eight scientific journals regarding the gender of the participants and reported that 65% of the articles referred to participants, of which 26% did not report any gender. In cases where gender was distinguished, 6% of the articles referred to female participants, 8% referred to male participants, and 60% referred to both female and male participants. Based on these results, the authors concluded that the gender effect was unclear in many studies. Wilson (2009) is a proponent of specifying gender in research (more about Wilson's work in the Section "men"). This specification is necessary to gain insight into gender-specific factors to obtain a better understanding of sexuality in people with an ID. In our research into sexuality and sexual health, we have made efforts to specify gender differences.

5.1 Women With Intellectual Disability

Noonan-Walsh and Heller (2002) concluded that gender has a specific influence on the health of people during their lives. A literature review

(Ouellette-Kuntz, 2005) into the health of people with ID showed that some attention is paid to the gynecological health of women, such as examinations for menopause, menstruation, Pap smears, mammography, and uterine tumors. Due to the lack of focus on women with an ID in research on other aspects of health and socioeconomic status, Noonan-Walsh and Heller focused on a number of topics beyond health that are important for females with an ID in their book. For example, in relation to sexuality, they examined sterilization, birth control, sexuality, parenthood, and risk and vulnerability. McCarthy (2001, 2002, 2009) has argued in favor of specific attention for research into the sexuality of females with an ID (McCarthy, Hunt, & Milne-Skillman, 2017). Support and assistance for females with ID are emphatically required because women are faced more frequently with sexual violence and abuse, their self-image is often poor, and they have little enjoyment from sex.

In general, women with an ID have a negative view of their own sexuality. These results were shown in a study involving 17 women with an ID (McCarthy, 2001). Most of these women did not see themselves as a sexual person, even though they were sexually active. For example, one individual (MC) told the interviewer (MM).

> *MC: I have no sexual feelings whatsoever.*
>
> *MM: But you do have sex, so is it something you want or is it something that just happens to you?*
>
> *MC: A rather lot of it is forced on me*
>
> ***McCarthy (2001, p. 199).***

According to McCarthy (2001), there are four important factors that contribute to the generally negative experiences with sex reported by women with an ID: (1) a lack of sexual autonomy, (2) the nature of the sexual activities that took place, (3) the fact that the activities are primarily experienced on a physical level, and (4) many experiences with sexual abuse.

Sexual autonomy means that you can decide for yourself what you want to do with whom, where, when, and how (WHO, 2015). To make these decisions, however, you must have certain knowledge and skills. For example, you must know what you like and do not like in terms of sex. Masturbation is one way to discover your own body and to determine what you like and do not like. Fewer women with an ID report having experience with masturbation than their peers without ID (McCarthy, 2001, 2009). For example, one participant (EY), told the interviewer (MM).

> *MM: Is it (masturbation) wrong for men and women?*
>
> *EY: For women because they can injure themselves. If they put their hand up the front and keep rubbing themselves, they might injure their vagina or something like that....*
>
> ***McCarthy (2001, p. 129)***

Another participant (MC) responded,

> *MM: Do you think women get sexual urges?*
>
> *MC: No.*
>
> *MM: Why not?*
>
> *MC: The only sexual urges a woman can have is if a fella takes her to have sex. Otherwise they haven't got any.*
>
> ***McCarthy (2001, p. 130)***

Masturbation is an important, but neglected, topic in sexual health for women with ID. The topic is mainly approached from a negative point of view. In the study of Bernert and Ogletree (2013) none of the 14 women reported to have experience with masturbation. Further, McCarthy (2001, p. 128) found that masturbation was a sensitive topic, stating, "Two women (of the 17 women) avoided the question completely... None of the women readily or confidently reported that they masturbated, despite." Masturbation by men is judged more positively by women with ID. For example, one woman stated, "...men do it a lot if they feel sexually inclined towards a woman and they can't get one, but for women it's not a good idea, even if they're in bed, because it doesn't prove anything and it's wrong to do it" (McCarthy, 2001, p. 129). McCarthy (2002) concludes that there is no reason to ascertain that women with ID really masturbate less than other women. She points out that women with ID find it uncomfortable to talk about this subject. It is essential that positive attention is given to masturbation, as for individuals who are not capable of having sex with others, masturbation offers an outlet and a way to experience sexuality.

In addition, knowledge and skills in terms of setting limits are important. The empowerment of people with ID is generally lower than people without disabilities, and women are even more vulnerable in this respect. Bernert (2011) interviewed 14 women with ID and reported that women had a strong sense of autonomy: "It's my life, not [theirs]." The women felt they were adult women. However, this sexual autonomy was often thwarted by their male sexual partners, by professional carers, or by family members. Bernert (2011, p. 134) reported: "In many ways, the women were not able to act autonomously without services or assistance from outsiders, and thus, assistance from outsiders was essential to the women's autonomy. This inverted relationship between autonomy and dependence held true for all of the women."

The sexual activities of women with an ID appear to be primarily focused on giving pleasure to men (McCarthy, 2001). Penetration (vaginal and anal sex) is at the top of the list, followed by the woman touching the penis or giving fellatio. At the bottom of the list is cunnilingus given by the man. Besides the usual focus on giving pleasure to the male sex partner, many women experience pain during sex, resulting in a frequently negative association with sex. Anal sex and oral sex (fellatio) were reported as the least favorite activities. One-third of the women indicated that they preferred to kiss and hug (McCarthy, 2001). As a result, the study by Bernert and Ogletree (2013), interviewing 14 women with ID, showed that abstinence is used as a strategy to avoid negative experiences such as pregnancy, STDs, coercion, and abuse. One participant stated, "I'm scared of it. It might hurt." She also wanted to avoid pregnancy and HIV, another reason she has said to "don't have sex." (in Bernert & Ogletree, 2013, p. 245). Another participant stated, "Well, I mean if you're not, if you're not very careful, you get trouble doin' things you're not suppose to do. Things like (sex)" (in Bernert & Ogletree, 2013, p. 245).

The knowledge and experiences of this group of women with ID was primarily focused on the physical level of sexuality. It appears that women primarily learn factual aspects (how to do something), and that no attention is paid to feelings such as pleasure, desire, and excitement. It also appears that men pay little attention to the woman's feelings during sex. Fitzgerald and Withers (2011) interviewed 10 women with ID about their sexuality and sexual identity. The women stated that they did not see themselves as sexual beings, but as passive with respect to sexuality. They felt that sexual activity should primarily focus on giving pleasure to the man and that it was not their task to participate actively in sexual activities. They did not experience any pleasure from these activities. The women considered themselves to be of little value. Fitzgerald and Withers (2011, p. 10) concluded:

> *The implicit messages given by the women throughout the interviews were that men were somehow better and more valuable than women, although paradoxically a number of women said that they worked harder than men. The women seemed to view men as being privileged in society without merit. They felt powerless in relation to men, and this was reflected in their accounts of sexual and financial exploitation.*

A literature review by McCarthy (2014) showed that the situation has not changed substantially during the past 10 years for women with an ID. As one staff member questioned, "When have they had an opportunity to have a positive experience? I mean, they're not educated about it. They don't have the right place to do it. So how are they going to see sex as positive?" (Bernert & Ogletree, 2013, p. 246). More recently, authors have urged a greater focus on the pleasurable aspects of sexuality: "...professionals providing services and education should emphasize sex positive messages that contribute to sexual self-efficacy, self-determination, and self-advocacy among women" (Bernert & Ogletree, 2013, p. 247). The sexual script that these women learn must include sexual expression, pleasure, and mutual exchange.

5.2 Men With Intellectual Disability

Research into the sexuality of males with an ID is frequently limited to two aspects: (1) the high risk of HIV or (2) being a perpetrator of sexual abuse/engaging in undesirable or problematic sexual behavior. Wilson (2009) denounced the lack of attention for the specific sexual health problems of males.

In a review of four international journals (Journal of Intellectual Disability Research, Journal of Applied Research in Intellectual Disabilities, American Journal on Mental Retardation, and Journal of Intellectual and Developmental Disability) focusing specifically on research involving people with an ID, Wilson (2009) studied the titles of articles published since 2000 that focused on males and females with ID. For males (search terms: "male, man, boy, or men") he found the following: 3 articles about "mental health"; 9 articles about "sexual matters" in which male sexuality was primarily presented in a problematic context; 9 articles about "health and well-being"; 10 articles about "crime/antisocial behavior," of which 6 were related to sexuality ("sexual abuse, sex offenders, sexually abusive behavior"); 8 articles about "language," and 6 articles on other topics. For purposes of comparison, the same study was conducted for females (search terms: "female, woman, girl or women"). He found 21 articles about "health and well-being"; 1 article about sexuality, in which women were victims of sexual abuse; 3 articles about "crime/antisocial behavior," and 12 articles about "other" topics. The differences in focus for males and females are striking. Furthermore, the negative approach to male sexuality is striking.

Another literature review (Ouellette-Kuntz, 2005) found that while there is attention paid to a part of the sexual health problems of females with an ID, no attention is paid to the specific sexual health problems of males, such as prostate screening and examination of testes. Hogg and Tuffrey-Wijne (2008) conducted a literature review on the incidence and prevalence of cancer in people with an ID. In the literature review, they reported significantly more cases of testicular cancer in males with a severe or very severe ID and in males with Down syndrome. Thus, they argued in favor of screening for gender-specific forms of cancer, both in males and females with an ID.

The problems experienced by men with an ID with respect to pleasurable and safe sex concern masturbation, among other aspects. The problems included a lack of understanding about how to masturbate, being unable to have an orgasm, masturbating inappropriately, or using objects for masturbation that are harmful (Cambridge, Beadle-Brown, Milne, Mansell, & Whelton, 2011; Van Doorn, van den Bogaard, & Embregts, 2014). For males with an ID, many of these problems can be traced back to a lack of knowledge, skills, and support.

In summary, it can be stated that education and support should focus on preventing problems such as unplanned pregnancies, sexual abuse, or STDs. However, it is also important to pay attention to the pleasurable and enjoyable aspects of sexuality. Masturbation, or solo sex, is a theme that deserves explicit attention for individuals with an ID. It is a way to explore one's own body and sexuality. In the case of women in particular, this exploration is not always taken for granted.

Finally, people with an ID often have little space to experiment sexually. This lack of experimentation is because the protective environment exerts control, resulting in little privacy. To develop sexually, however, room for experimentation is essential. A balance must be struck between protecting someone with an ID and offering them the possibility to develop sexually. In addition, more research is needed into the gender-specific health problems and needs of males and females with an ID.

6. SEXUAL DIVERSITY

Sexual diversity refers to "the full range of sexuality which includes all aspects of sexual attraction, behavior, identity, expression, orientation, relationships and response. It refers to all aspects of humans as sexual beings" according to the International Planned Parenthood Federation (2008, p. 66). Sexual diversity also occurs in people with ID. However, very little is known about the extent to which the sexual diversity differs relative to the general population. For the time being, there is no reason to assume that there is a substantial difference between these groups. People with ID experience additional prejudices and discrimination from other people with ID as well as from people without ID. Further, lesbian, gay, bisexual, or transgender (LGBT) individuals with ID have few opportunities to make social acquaintances (Abbott, 2013; Abbott & Burns, 2007; Abbott & Howarth, 2005, 2007; Fraley, Mona, & Theodore, 2007; McCann, Lee, & Brown, 2016; Stoffelen et al., 2013, 2017).

6.1 Prevalence

Estimating the number of LGBT people with an ID is not a simple task. To estimate the number of homosexual or bisexual people without ID, a "self-identified" criterion is used (Bakker & Wijsen, 2013). Savin-Williams and Cohen (2007) distinguish seven stages in the sexual development of LGBT youths: (1) feeling different; (2) attraction to same sex; (3) doubting own heterosexuality; (4) sex with someone of the same gender; (5) self-identification; (6) coming-out; and (7) acceptance. A certain level of cognitive ability is needed for this self-identification process (Vanwesenbeeck, 2006). However, for many people with an ID, especially if the ID is moderate, severe, or very severe, self-identification may not be possible (Kok et al., 2009). The lack of research into the prevalence of sexual diversity among people with an ID is therefore not particularly surprising (Löfgren-Mårtenson, 2009; Noonan & Taylor Gomez, 2011). Precisely because of their disability, many people with an ID do not identify themselves as LGBT and/or they experience sexuality in a completely different way (Kok et al., 2009; Stoffelen et al., 2013).

McCann et al. (2016, p. 50) conclude in their review of the literature concerning ID and LGBT: "…some are LGBT and some men with ID have sex with other men."

6.2 Scarce Research

Research into sexual diversity among people with ID is scarce (Fraley et al., 2007). Almost no research is available concerning experiences with same-sex relationships for people with an ID (Abbott, 2013). Of the research that has been performed, it is primarily from the male perspective, leading to great underrepresentation of women with an ID (Abbott & Howarth, 2005, 2007; Abbott, 2013; Cambridge, 1997; Cambridge & Mellan, 2000; Stoffelen et al., 2013). The perspective of lesbian, bisexual, or transgender women is absent in virtually all research; these women appear to be invisible (Bernert & Ogletree, 2013; Burns & Davies, 2011; Duke, 2011; McCann et al., 2016; McCarthy, 2001). In a study conducted by Abbott and Howarth (2005), the authors attempted to better understand the experiences of gay, lesbian, and bisexual men and women, through interviews with 71 staff members, 9 women, and 11 men with ID. They concluded, "It was relatively easy to find men to interview but we struggled to find nine lesbian and bisexual women with ID."

6.3 Prejudice and Stigmatization

The few studies that have been conducted into individuals with an ID who are LGBT have noted the prejudice and stigmatization experienced by this group. Individuals with an ID who are homosexual experience prejudice and intimidation from the outside world. Because they have an ID and are homosexual, they are doubly stigmatized; this double stigma is referred to as a "layered" stigma (Crocker, 2005; Duke, 2011; Goffman, 1963; Löfgren-Mårtenson, 2009; Meyer, 2003). Prejudice and discrimination limit the possibilities to participate in society and the opportunities to develop friendships (Hall, 2010). For example, individuals with an ID who are LGBT experience bullying, exclusion, or discrimination by others (Abbott, 2013; Burns & Davies, 2011; Duke, 2011; Leutar & Mihoković, 2007; Löfgren-Mårtenson, 2004, 2009; Stoffelen et al., 2013). These individuals are often bullied at work or when they go to cafés or nightclubs (Duke, 2011; Stoffelen et al., 2013). They are also stigmatized by homosexuals without ID (Stoffelen et al., 2013). In the "homosexual world" people with an ID find themselves at the bottom of the "gay pecking order" due to their lack of social contacts and money (Thompson, Bryson, & de Castell, 2001).

Further, people with and without IDs often have prejudices and are negative about homosexuality. As such, young people with an ID sometimes internalize the homophobic and heterosexual attitude of their carers, teachers, parents, and coworkers (Duke, 2011). As a further result of this stigmatization, individuals with an ID who are LGBT are often reluctant to tell others that they are homosexual (Stoffelen et al., 2013). For example, one individual stated, " I'm afraid how they will react. At my work...when I say I like girls...they don't want to sit next to me" (female, aged 29, in Stoffelen et al., 2013, p. 261).

In response to prejudice and stigma, individuals with an ID are afraid to be themselves in public. They often find it difficult to be assertive about their sexuality (Abbott & Howarth, 2005, 2007; Cambridge & Mellan, 2000; Duke, 2011; Stoffelen et al. 2013). For example, one individual stated, "If I get new work, I will definitely keep my mouth shut..." (male, aged 51, in Stoffelen et al., 2013, p. 261). And another individual said,

> *They hollered at me and called me a homo. That wasn't nice. They were disciplined by the boss. Homos are people too. They are just normal people*
>
> ***Male, aged 53, in Stoffelen et al., 2013, p. 261.***

6.4 Social Contacts

Many people meet their future partners at work, through friends, or during other social contacts. For individuals with an ID who are LGBT, it is more difficult to meet others and their social networks are often very limited. The chance that they will make contact with another individual who is LGBT is small (Abbott & Howarth, 2005; Fraley et al., 2007; Stoffelen et al., 2013). In the Netherlands, occasional meetups for individuals with an ID who are LGBT (COC-cafes) are held, but the required travel is a problem for many people, especially those who live outside the big cities (Stoffelen et al., 2013). Unfortunately, transportation is always a problem if you have an ID (Shakespeare, 2006). This transportation problem is unfortunate because it is crucial to meet others, for example, to experiment with relationships, gain experience, develop a positive self-image, and become empowered (Duke, 2011). To overcome the issues with transportation, Fraley et al. (2007) referred to the possibilities offered by the Internet, although the experiences are not always positive (Stoffelen et al., 2013, 2017), as one participant noted:

> *I'm now looking on dating sites. I've registered for several: Badoo, Tinder. I'm not really looking, because looking doesn't help… but I did have contact with someone for years. And now I want more. It was a faker, it was a man. On Facebook, it looked like a pretty woman…I felt awful about this for a long time. It kept me awake. It was miserable.*
>
> ***Female, aged 23, in Stoffelen et al., 2017.***

Another individual stated,

> *Of course I would like to have a relationship sometime, but I'm not looking specifically. If you force yourself to look, then you find the weirdest types. You have to wait for someone you really like. I don't know many people, hardly any women…I'm the only woman in my group of friends*
>
> ***Female, aged 25, in Stoffelen et al., 2017.***

And finally,

> *I have my eye on a girl. She lives a few streets away. But she also has problems with anxiety, so neither of us dares to make contact. It could take a long time*
>
> ***Female, aged 25, in Stoffelen et al., 2017.***

6.5 Support

Although research into the specific health problems of LGBT people with an ID is scarce (Fraley et al., 2007), some research indicates that LGBT individuals with an ID have an increased risk of depression, anxiety, drug use, loneliness, sexual problems, and sexual violence (Bakker & Wijsen, 2013; Clarke, Ellis, Peel, & Riggs, 2010; de Graaf, Bakker, & Wijsen, 2014; Duke, 2011). Thus, when it comes to sexual diversity and supporting people with an ID three aspects are vitally important: (1) providing information, education, and training; (2) providing positive support; and (3) providing accessible information.

Information, education, and training about sexuality are crucial; not only for people with an ID but also for their carers, family members; and others who represent their interests. The informational material should focus especially on sexual diversity and themes such as prevention of HIV/AIDS, attention to homophobia, and gaining access to the LGBT community (Duke, 2011; Fraley et al., 2007; Löfgren-Mårtenson, 2009; Noonan & Taylor Gomez, 2011; Stoffelen et al. 2013; Thompson, 2007). Finally, providing support and role models is important for the development of a positive identity (Abbott, 2013; Abbott & Howarth, 2005; Duke, 2011;

Löfgren-Mårtenson, 2009; Noonan & Taylor Gomez, 2011; Stoffelen et al., 2013). "It's probably also pretty hard for them to understand it themselves, because one knows how difficult it is for other homosexuals to be accepted and so you know it must be even more difficult for mentally challenged people to understand and accept themselves..." (staff member in Löfgren-Mårtenson, 2009, p. 23–24).

Accessible information about LGBT sexuality by means of good, easy-to-read books, and websites is needed for people with an ID (Duke, 2011; Löfgren-Mårtenson, 2009; Stoffelen et al., 2013). Löfgren-Mårtenson (2009) interviewed people with ID, parents, and staff members to identify and describe the variety of sexual expression, such as homosexuality and bisexuality. She describes in her article the situation in Sweden, "Easy-to-read literature designed for people with ID in Sweden consists of a single book about homosexuality, and it is about male homosexuality. Books about same-sex sexuality among women do not exist at all, even if they form part of the plot of at least one recent easy-to-read book" (Löfgren-Mårtenson, 2009, pp. 25–26).

In summary, it can be stated that attention for sexual diversity among people with an ID is still a neglected aspect. These individuals are faced with the double stigma of having both an ID and a different sexual preference. This group has a great need for specific support. In research, women are greatly underrepresented.

7. SUPPORT FOR SEXUOLOGICAL PROBLEMS

Greenwood and Wilkinson (2013) conducted a literature review related to aspects of sexual health of women with ID, including sexual health care. They noticed a lack of "primary care-focused research and practice guidelines for the sexual health care of adult women with intellectual disabilities" (Greenwood & Wilkinson, 2013, p. 1).

From research into the sexual problems of women with an ID, the following aspects have emerged: lack of knowledge and skills, negative experiences, no understanding of one's own sexual desires, pain during intercourse, and dissatisfaction with their sex partner, the absence of a partner, and no access to help (Greenwood & Wilkinson, 2013; Van Doorn et al., 2014). Research involving men has also shown inadequate knowledge and skills, dissatisfaction with a partner (or the lack of partner) for sexual contact or a sexual relationship, excessive or inappropriate masturbation, inappropriate touching and/or approaching others, and erection problems (Van Doorn et al., 2014).

For problems with sexuality, people with an ID can contact sexologists. In the Netherlands, sexologists can be employed in residential settings for people with an ID. Most of the referrals to the sexologists have something to do with the embarrassment of the carers when faced with the sexual health needs of residents (Manders et al., 2010). These sexologists collaborate within the national sexology platform working with people with mild ID (Landelijk Platform Netwerk Seksuologie en LVB). The platform endeavors to disseminate knowledge on diagnostics, research, and organization. Using the national sexology platform, Van Zenderen and Hehenkamp (2015) investigated the reasons for referral of 154 clients (67% male, 23% female; 15.5% with moderate ID, 54.5% with mild ID, and 14% with borderline ID). The main reasons for referral were sexual abuse and/or violence, sexual dissatisfaction, and inappropriate sexual behavior. More sexological support is required for people with ID. In addition, we need research beyond just the Netherlands.

8. CONCLUSION

Just as those without ID, individuals with ID have sexual needs, expressions, drives, and desires. Individuals with an ID may also differ from the general population of people without an ID in certain aspects. These aspects, therefore, require extra attention.

Those who provide support to people with ID should have insight into the differences in sexual development experienced by individuals with ID and they must be knowledgeable as to which aspects are unusual. As in the general population, asexuality is present but it is not the norm. Rather, people with a mild ID want to have relationships and sexual experiences. Although very little research has been conducted into the sexuality of people with a severe ID, it is believed that all individuals want to experience relationships.

To address the diverse nature of individuals with an ID, it is important to take account of their learning difficulties and limitations in adaptive skills when providing sex education to this population. Such difficulties and limitations may make it more difficult for individuals with an ID to understand and remember information. It is therefore important to adapt the sex education curriculum accordingly. For example, repeating information and practicing skills a number of times are essential activities for this group.

Research into the development of sex education material has shown that too much emphasis is still placed on talking about individuals with an ID instead of talking with the individuals with an ID. Engaging in dialogue with the individuals with an ID is essential when approaching the "loaded" topic of sex. It is essential to determine the individual's perspective on sexuality, while trying to think and act outside one's own normative framework.

The positive aspects of sexuality should also be given attention. At the same time, the associated hazards should also be taken into account, such as sexual abuse, unplanned pregnancy, and STDs. Entering into and maintaining relationships is a problematic area for people with an ID, especially where sexual relationships are concerned. Education on these aspects must begin early and be attuned to the possibilities of the target group.

Masturbation, or solo sex, should also be addressed in the informative material. Especially among females, there is often a lack of experience with masturbation and orgasm. Males, in contrast, may engage in masturbation in an unhealthy or inappropriate way. Specific attention for pleasurable and healthy masturbation is therefore required.

Many women with an ID do not experience enjoyable sex with a partner. Rather, during sexual activity the focus is primarily on giving pleasure to the male sex partner. Attention to the satisfaction of the woman and how she can have an orgasm is therefore important. Further, more research into gender-specific sexual health in women and men with ID is needed to better understand their specific needs and the factors that play a role in this process. Research is also needed to change the often prevailing gender stereotypes about ID and sexuality.

Finally, sexual diversity is also present in people with an ID. Consequently, they are faced with a double stigma: they not only have an ID but also a different sexual preference. More attention for this group and providing specific support to them is important to improve their quality of life and sexual health.

As stated previously, this chapter is primarily about the sexual health of individuals with a mild ID. Little research has been conducted into the sexuality of people with a severe or very severe ID. Almost no data on the sexuality of these groups are available. When using a term "intellectual disability" or "learning disabilities" and descriptions of the degree of ID it is important to keep in mind the important statement preceding these definitions that people with IDs are "people first." Supporting or rejecting the sexual needs and wishes of people with IDs reflects the attitudes, values, and beliefs of our society and deeply affects their lives.

REFERENCES

AAIDD. (2008). *Sexuality. Position statement of AAIDD and the arc.* Washington: AAIDD.

Abbott, D. (2013). Nudge, nudge, wink, wink: Love, sex and gay men with intellectual disabilities — A helping hand or a human right? *Journal of Intellectual Disability Research, 57*, 1079—1087. http://dx.doi.org/10.1111/j.1365-2788.2012.01642.x.

Abbott, D., & Burns, J. (2007). What's love got to do with it?: Experiences of lesbian, gay, and bisexual people with intellectual disabilities in the United Kingdom and views of the staff who support them. *Sexuality Research & Social Policy: A Journal of the NSRC, 4*(1), 27—39. http://dx.doi.org/10.1525/srsp.2007.4.1.27.

Abbott, D., & Howarth, J. (2005). *Secret loves, hidden lives? Exploring issues for people with learning difficulties who are gay, lesbian or bisexual.* Bristol: The Policy Press.

Abbott, D., & Howarth, J. (2007). Still off-limits? Staff views on supporting gay, lesbian and bisexual people with intellectual disabilities to develop sexual and intimate relationships? *Journal of Applied Research in Intellectual Disabilities, 20*, 116—126. http://dx.doi.org/10.1111/j.1468-3148.2006.00312.x.

American Psychiatric Association. (2013). *Diagnostic and statistical manual of mental disorders* (5th ed.). Arlington, VA: American Psychiatric Association.

Bakker, B., & Wijsen, C. (2013). *Wat maakt het verschil? Diversiteit in de seksuele gezondheid van LHBT's. Een verkenning* [*What makes the difference? Diversity in the sexual health of LGBT. An exploration*]. Utrecht: Rutgers WPF.

Bankras, M., van Loon, L., & Reijenga, R. (2011). *Williams syndrome. Samenvatting van een referaat* [*Williams syndrome. Summary paper*]. Rotterdam: Erasmus Medical Centre.

Bernert, D. (2011). Sexuality and disability in the lives of women with intellectual disabilities. *Sexuality and Disability, 29*, 129—141. http://dx.doi.org/10.1007/s11195-010-9190-4.

Bernert, D. J., & Ogletree, R. J. (2013). Women with intellectual disabilities talk about their perceptions of sex. *Journal of Intellectual Disability Research, 57*, 240—249. http://dx.doi.org/10.1111/j.1365-2788.2011.01529.x.

Beumer, S., & Bevers, M. (2014). *Down syndroom. Samenvatting van een referaat* [*Down syndrome. Summary paper*]. Rotterdam: Erasmus Medical Centre.

de Bruijn, J., Buntinx, W., & Twint, B. (2014). *Verstandelijke beperking: Definitie en context* [*Intellectual disability: Definition and context*]. Amsterdam: Uitgeverij SWP.

Burns, J., & Davies, D. (2011). Same-sex relationships and women with intellectual disabilities. *Journal of Applied Research in Intellectual Disabilities, 24*, 351—360. http://dx.doi.org/10.1111/j.1468-3148.2010.00609.x.

Cambridge, P. (1997). How far to gay? The politics of HIV in learning disability. *Disability & Society, 12*, 427—453.

Cambridge, P., Beadle-Brown, J., Milne, A., Mansell, J., & Whelton, B. (2011). Patterns of risk in adult protection referrals for sexual abuse and people with intellectual disability. *Journal of Applied Research in Intellectual Disabilities, 24*, 118—132. http://dx.doi.org/10.1111/j.1468-3148.2010.00574.x.

Cambridge, P., & Mellan, B. (2000). Reconstructing the sexuality of men with learning disabilities: Empirical evidence and theoretical interpretations of need. *Disability and Society, 15*, 293—311.

Chiurazzi, P., & Pirozzi, F. (2016). Advances in understanding - genetic basis of intellectual disability. *F1000 Research*. http://dx.doi.org/10.12688/f1000research.7134.1. Faculty Rev-599.

Christian, L., Stinson, J., & Dotson, L. A. (2001). Staff values regarding the sexual expression of women with developmental disabilities. *Sexuality and Disability, 19*(4), 283–291. http://dx.doi.org/10.1023/A:1017957409670.

Clarke, V., Ellis, S. J., Peel, E., & Riggs, D. W. (2010). *Lesbian, gay, bisexual, trans & queer psychology. An introduction*. Cambridge: Cambridge University Press.

Crocker, J. (2005). De sociale psychologie van stigmatisering [The social psychology of stigma]. *Tijdschrift voor Seksuologie, 29*, 4–10.

Cuskelly, M., & Bryde, R. (2004). Attitudes towards the sexuality of adults with an intellectual disability: Parents, support staff, and a community sample. *Journal of Intellectual & Developmental Disability, 29*(3), 255–264. http://dx.doi.org/10.1080/13668250412331285136.

Demirdas, S., Ganzevoort, T., & Fischer, S. (2016). *Foetaal alcohol syndroom (FAS) en Fetal alcohol spectrum disorder (FASD). Samenvatting [Fetal alcohol syndrome (FAS) and Fetal Alcohol Syndrome Disorder (FASD). Summary paper]*. Rotterdam: Erasmus Medical Centre.

Duke, T. S. (2011). Lesbian, gay, bisexual and transgender youth with disabilities: A meta-synthesis. *Journal of LHBT Youth, 8*, 1–52. http://dx.doi.org/10.1080/19361653.2011.519181.

Dykens, E. M., & Hodapp, R. M. (1999). Behavioural phenotypes: Towards new understandings of people with developmental disabilities. *Psychiatric and Behavioural Disorders in Developmental Disabilities and Mental Retardation*, 96–108.

Eastgate, G., Van Driel, M. L., Lennox, N., & Scheermeyer, E. (2011). Women with intellectual disabilities. A study of sexuality, sexual abuse and protection skills. *Australian Family Physician, 40*(4), 226–229.

Egemo-Helm, K. R., Miltenberger, R. G., Knudson, P., Finstrom, N., Jostad, C., & Johnson, B. (2007). An evaluation of in situ training to teach sexual abuse prevention skills to women with mental retardation. *Behavioral Interventions, 22*, 99–119. http://dx.doi.org/10.1002/bin.234.

Evans, D. S., McGuire, B. E., Healy, E., & Carley, S. N. (2009). Sexuality and personal relationship for people with an intellectual disability. Part II: Staff and family carer perspectives. *Journal of Intellectual Disability Research, 53*(11), 913–921. http://dx.doi.org/10.1111/j.1365-2788.2009.01202.x.

Fitzgerald, C., & Withers, P. (2011). 'I don't know what a proper woman means': What women with intellectual disabilities think about sex, sexuality and themselves. *British Journal of Learning Disabilities, 41*, 5–12.

Fraley, S. S., Mona, L. R., & Theodore, P. S. (2007). The sexual lives of lesbian, gay and bisexual people with disabilities: Psychological perspectives. *Sexuality Research and Social Policy, 4*, 15–27. http://dx.doi.org/10.1525/srsp.2007.4.1.15.

Fyson, R., & Kitson, D. (2010). Human rights and social wrongs: Issues in safeguarding adults with learning disabilities. Practice. *Social Work in Action, 22*(5), 309–320. http://dx.doi.org/10.1080/09503153.2010.517831.

Gilmore, L., & Cuskelly, M. (2014). Vulnerability to loneliness in people with intellectual disability: An explanatory model. *Journal of Policy and Practice in Intellectual Disabilities, 11*(3), 192–199. http://dx.doi.org/10.1111/jppi.12089.

Goffman, E. (1963). *Stigma. Notes on the management of spoiled identity*. New York: Simon & Schuster Inc.

de Graaf, H., Bakker, B. H. W., & Wijsen, C. (2014). *Een wereld van verschil. De seksuele gezondheid van LHBT's in Nederland 2013 [A world of difference. The sexual health of LGBT in the Netherlands in 2013]*. Utrecht: Rutgers WPF.

Greenwood, N. W., & Wilkinson, J. (2013). Sexual and reproductive health care for women with intellectual disabilities: A primary care perspective. *International Journal of Family Medicine*. http://dx.doi.org/10.1155/2013/642472.

Hall, S. A. (2010). *The social inclusion of young adults with intellectual disabilities: A phenomenology of their experiences*. Lincoln, NE: University of Nebraska.

Hayashi, M., Arakida, M., & Ohashi, K. (2011). The effectiveness of a sex education program facilitating social skills for people with intellectual disability in Japan. *Journal of Intellectual & Developmental Disability, 36*, 11–19. http://dx.doi.org/10.3109/13668250.2010.549463.

Healy, E., McGuire, B. E., Evans, D. S., & Carley, S. N. (2009). Sexuality and personal relationships for people with an intellectual disability. Part I: Service-user perspectives. *Journal of Intellectual Disability Research, 53*, 905–912. http://dx.doi.org/10.1111/j.1365-2788.2009.01203.x.

Heestermans, M., van den Boogaard, K., & Embregts, P. (2015). *Gezegd of gezwegen: Diagnostiek bij seksueel misbruik van en door mensen met een verstandelijke beperking* [*Diagnosing sexual abuse in people with an intellectual disability*]. Apeldoorn: Dichterbij Kennisn@.

Hendriks, A., & Legemaate, J. (2009). *Thematic legal study on mental health and fundamental rights*. The Netherlands: European Union Agency for Fundamental Rights (FRA).

Hendrikx, A., & Mulder, A. (2016). *Angelman en Prader-Willi syndroom. Samenvatting referaat* [*Angelman and Prader-Willi syndrome. Summary paper*]. Rotterdam: Erasmus Medical Centre.

Hickson, L., Khemka, I., Golden, H., & Chatzistyli, A. (2008). Profiles of women who have mental retardation with and without a documented history of abuse. *American Journal on Mental Retardation, 113*(2), 133–142. http://dx.doi.org/10.1352/0895-8017(2008)113[133:POWWHM]2.0.CO;2.

Hodapp, R. M., & Dykens, E. M. (2004). Studying behavioral phenotypes: Issues, benefits, challenges. In E. Emerson, C. Hatton, T. Thompson, & T. R. Parmenter (Eds.), *The international handbook of applied research in intellectual disabilities* (pp. 203–211). West Sussex: John Wiley & Sons Ltd.

Hodes, M. W. (2017). *Testing the effect of parenting support for people with intellectual disabilities and borderline intellectual functioning*. Apeldoorn: Drukmotief.

Hogg, J., & Tuffrey-Wijne, I. (2008). Cancer and intellectual disability: A review of some key contextual issues. *British Journal of Learning Disabilities, 21*(6), 509–518.

Hollomotz, A. (2008). 'May we please have sex tonight?' – People with learning difficulties pursuing privacy in residential group settings. *British Journal of Learning Disabilities, 37*, 91–97. http://dx.doi.org/10.1111/j.1468-3156.2008.00512.x.

Hollomotz, A. (2011). *Learning difficulties and sexual vulnerability. A social approach*. London: Jessica Kingsley Publishers.

Holm, V. A., Cassidy, S. B., Butler, M. G., Hanchett, J. M., Greenswag, L. R., Whitman, B. Y., & Greenberg, F. (1993). Prader-willi syndrome: Consensus diagnostic criteria. *Pediatrics, 91*(2), 398–402.

Howard-Barr, E. M., Rienzo, B. A., Pigg, R. M., & James, D. (2005). Teacher beliefs, professional preparation, and practices regarding exceptional students and sexuality education. *Journal of School Health, 75*, 99–104.

Hubert, J. (2009). *The realities of life for people with severe and profound intellectual disabilities and mental health problems*. Maastricht: Maastricht University.

Ignagni, E., Fudge Schormans, A., Liddiard, K., & Runswick-Cole, K. (2016). 'Some people are not allowed to love': Intimate citizenship in the lives of people labelled with intellectual disabilities. *Disability & Society, 31*(1), 131–135. http://dx.doi.org/10.1080/09687599.2015.1136148.

International Planned Parenthood Federation. (2008). *Sexual diversity tool kit. 5. Glossary*. New York: IPPF. https://www.ippfwhr.org/sites/default/files/uploaded_documents/SexualDiversityToolKit_Section5.pdf.

Kalthoff, H. (2015). *Verstandelijk beperkte ouders. Wat betekent het voor een kind om verstandelijk beperkte ouders te hebben [Mentally disabled parents. What does it mean for a child to have parents with intellectual disabilities?]*. Utrecht: Nederland Jeugdinstituut.

Kelly, G., Crowley, H., & Hamilton, C. (2009). Rights, sexuality and relationships in Ireland: 'It'd be nice to be kind of trusted'. *British Journal of Learning Disabilities, 37*, 308–315. http://dx.doi.org/10.1111/j.1468-3156.2009.00587.x.

Khemka, I., Hickson, L., & Reynolds, G. (2005). Evaluation of a decision-making curriculum designed to empower women with mental retardation to resist abuse. *American Journal on Mental Retardation, 110*(3), 193–204. http://dx.doi.org/10.1352/0895-8017(2005)110<193:EOADCD>2.0.CO;2.

Kok, G., Maassen, R., Maaskant, M., & Curfs, L. (2009). Zorgverleners over seksualiteit van mensen met verstandelijke beperkingen; een kwalitatief onderzoek [Caregivers about sexuality on people with intellectual disabilities; a qualitative study]. *Tijdschrift voor Seksuologie, 33*, 199–206.

Kraijer, D. W., & Plas, J. J. (2007). *Handboek psychodiagnostiek en beperkte begaafdheid. Classificatie, test-, schaal- en vragenlijstgebruik [Handbook psychodiagnostics and limited giftedness. Classification, test, scale and questionnaire use]*. Amsterdam: Harcourt Book Publishers.

Lafferty, A., McConkey, R., & Simpson, A. (2012). Reducing the barriers to relationships and sexuality education for persons with intellectual disabilities. *Journal of Intellectual Disabilities, 16*, 29–43.

Lesseliers, J. (1999). A right to sexuality? *British Journal of Learning Disabilities, 27*, 137–140.

Leutar, Z., & Mihoković, M. (2007). Level of knowledge about sexuality of people with mental disabilities. *Sexuality and Disability, 25*, 93–109. http://dx.doi.org/10.1007/s11195-007-9046-8.

Levy, H., & Packman, W. (2004). Sexual abuse prevention for individuals with mental retardation: Considerations for genetic counselors. *Journal of Genetic Counseling, 13*, 189–205. http://dx.doi.org/10.1023/B: JOGC.0000028158.79395.1e.

de Ligt, J., Willemsen, M., van Bon, B. W. M., Kleefstra, T., Yntema, H. G., Kroes, T., … Vissers, L. E. (2012). Diagnostic exome sequencing in persons with severe intellectual disability. *The New England Journal of Medicine, 367*(20), 1921–1929. http://dx.doi.org/10.1056/NEJMoa1206524.

Llewellyn, G., Traustadóttir, R., McConnell, D., & Sigurjónsdóttir, H. B. (2010). *Parents with intellectual disabilities. Past, present and futures*. Chichester, UK: John Wiley & Sons Ltd.

Löfgren-Mårtenson, L. (2004). 'May I?' about sexuality and love in the new generation with intellectual disabilities. *Sexuality and Disability, 22*, 197–207. http://dx.doi.org/10.1023/B: SEDI.0000039062.73691.cb.

Löfgren-Mårtenson, L. (2009). The invisibility of young homosexual women and men with intellectual disabilities. *Sexuality and Disability*, 7, 21–26. http://dx.doi.org/10.1007/s11195-008-9101-0.

Löfgren-Mårtenson, L. (2012). "I want to do it right!" A pilot study of Swedish sex education and young people with intellectual disabilities. *Sexuality and Disability, 30*, 209–225. http://dx.doi.org/10.1007/s11195-011-9239-z.

Manders, S., Stoffelen, J., Kedde, H., van Zelst, N., Kok, G., & Curfs, L. (2010). Seksuele problemen bij mensen met een verstandelijke beperking. Het ontwikkelen van een registratiesysteem ten behoeve van de seksuologische hulpverlening aan mensen met een verstandelijke beperking [Sexual problems in people with intellectual disability. The development of a recording system for the purpose of sex counseling for people with learning disabilities]. *Tijdschrift voor Seksuologie, 34*, 211–217.

Maulik, P. K., Mascarenhas, M. N., Mathers, C. D., Dua, T., & Saxena, S. (2011). Prevalence of intellectual disability. *Research in Developmental Disabilities, 32*(2), 419–436. http://dx.doi.org/10.1016/j.ridd.2010.12.018.

McCabe, M. P. (1999). Sexual knowledge, experience and feelings among people with disability. *Sexuality and Disability, 17*, 157–170. http://dx.doi.org/10.1023/A:1021476418440.

McCabe, M. P., Cummins, R. A., & Deeks, A. A. (1999). Construction and psychometric properties of sexuality scales: Sex knowledge, experience and needs scales for people with intellectual disabilities (SexKen-ID), people with physical disabilities (SexKen-PD) and the general population (SexKen-GP). *Research in Developmental Disabilities, 20*, 241–254. http://dx.doi.org/10.1016/S0891-4222(99)00007-4.

McCann, E., Lee, R., & Brown, M. (2016). The experiences and support needs of people with intellectual disabilities who identify as LGBT: A review of the literature. *Research in Developmental Disabilities, 57*, 39–53. http://dx.doi.org/10.1016/j.ridd.2016.06.013.

McCarthy, M. (2001). *Sexuality and women with learning disabilities*. London and Philadelphia: Jessica Kingsley Publishers.

McCarthy, M. (2002). Sexuality. In P. Noonan Walsh, & T. Heller (Eds.), *Health of women with intellectual disabilities* (pp. 90–103). Oxford: Blackwell Publishing Company.

McCarthy, M. (2009). Contraception and women with intellectual disabilities. *Journal of Applied Research in Intellectual Disabilities, 22*, 363–369. http://dx.doi.org/10.1111/j.1468-3148.2008.00464.x.

McCarthy, M. (2014). Women with intellectual disability: Their sexual lives in the 21st century. *Journal of Intellectual & Developmental Disability, 39*, 124–131. http://dx.doi.org/10.3109/13668250.2014.894963.

McCarthy, M., Hunt, S., & Milne-Skillman, K. (2017). 'I know it was every week, but I can't be sure if it was every day: Domestic violence and women with learning disabilities. *Journal of Applied Research in Intellectual Disabilities, 30*(2), 269–282. http://dx.doi.org/10.1111/jar.12237.

McGuire, B. E., & Bayley, A. A. (2011). Relationships, sexuality and decision-making capacity in people with an intellectual disability. *Current Opinion in Psychiatry, 24*, 398–402. http://dx.doi.org/10.1097/YCO.0b013e328349bbcb.

Meyer, I. H. (2003). Prejudice, social stress, and mental health in lesbian, gay and bisexual populations: Conceptual issues and research evidence. *Psychological Bulletin, 129*, 674–697. http://dx.doi.org/10.1037/0033-2909.129.5.674.

Miltenberger, R. G., Roberts, J. A., Ellingson, S., Galensky, T., Rapp, J. T., Long, E. S., & Lumley, V. A. (1999). Training and generalization of sexual abuse prevention skills for women with mental retardation. *Journal of Applied Behavior Analysis, 32*, 385–388. http://dx.doi.org/10.1901/jaba.1999.32-385.

Ministerie van Volksgezondheid Welzijn en Sport. (2004). *Anticonceptie voor verstandelijk gehandicapten* [*Contraception for the mentally disabled*]. kenmerk IBE/E-2472312, Den Haag: 29 April 2004.

Ministerie van Volksgezondheid Welzijn en Sport. (2006). *Brief aan de staatssecretaris van volksgezondheid, welzijn en sport* [*Letter to the Minister of health, welfare and sport*]. Den Haag: Tweede Kamer der Staten-Generaal, 2005–2006, 30 300 XVI, nr. 125.

Murphy, G. H., & O'Callaghan, A. (2004). Capacity of adults with intellectual disabilities to consent to sexual relationships. *Psychological Medicine, 34*, 1347–1357. http://dx.doi.org/10.1017/S0033291704001941.

Noonan, A., & Taylor Gomez, M. (2011). Who's missing? Awareness of lesbian, gay, bisexual and transgender people with intellectual disability. *Sexuality and Disability, 29*, 175–180. http://dx.doi.org/10.1007/s11195-010-9175-3.

Noonan-Walsh, P., & Heller, T. (2002). *Health of women with intellectual disabilities*. Oxford: Blackwell Publishing.

Nussbaum, M. C. (2014). *Mogelijkheden scheppen. Een nieuwe benadering van de menselijke ontwikkeling* [*Creating capabilities. The human development approach*]. Amsterdam: Ambo/Anthos uitgevers.

O'Callaghan, A. C., & Murphy, G. H. (2007). Sexual relationships in adults with intellectual disabilities: Understanding the law. *Journal of Intellectual Disability Research, 51*(3), 197–206. http://dx.doi.org/10.1111/j.1365-2788.2006.00857.x.

Ouellette-Kuntz, H. (2005). Understanding health disparities and inequities faced by individuals with intellectual disabilities. *Journal of Applied Research in Intellectual Disabilities, 18*(2), 113–121. http://dx.doi.org/10.1111/j.1468-3148.2005.00240.x.

Pahl, R. (2000). *On friendship*. Cambridge: Polity.

Peters, C. M., & Safi, M. (2012). Fragile X syndroom. *Samenvatting van een referaat*. Rotterdam: Erasmus Medical Centre.

Porter, C. L., Christian, L., & Poling, A. (2003). Research brief: Some data concerning the reporting of participants gender in the mental retardation literature. *Mental Retardation, 41*(2), 75–77. http://dx.doi.org/10.1352/0047-6765(2003)041<0075:RBSDCT>2.0.CO;2.

Rapport commissie Samson. (2012). *Omringd door zorg, toch niet veilig: Seksueel misbruik van door de overheid uit huis geplaatste kinderen, 1945 tot heden* [*Surrounded by care, still not safe*]. Amsterdam: Boom.

Reiter, S., Bryen, D. N., & Shachar, I. (2007). Adolescents with intellectual disabilities as victims of abuse. *Journal of Intellectual Disabilities, 11*(4), 371–387. http://dx.doi.org/10.1177/1744629507084602.

Rex, A. R., & Preus, M. (1982). A diagnostic index for down syndrome. *A Diagnostic Index for Down Syndrome, 100*(6), 903–906. http://dx.doi.org/10.1016/S0022-3476(82)80509-X.

Rohleder, P. (2010). Educators' ambivalence and managing anxiety in providing sex education for people with learning disabilities. Psychodynamic practice: Individuals. *Groups and Organisations, 16*, 165–182. http://dx.doi.org/10.1080/14753631003688100.

Rohleder, P., Braathen, S., Swartz, L., & Eide, A. H. (2009). HIV/AIDS and disability in Southern Africa: A review of relevant literature. *Disability and Rehabilitation, 31*, 51–59. http://dx.doi.org/10.1080/09638280802280585.

Savin-Williams, R. C., & Cohen, K. M. (2007). Development of same-sex attracted youth. In I. H. Meyer, & M. E. Northridge (Eds.), *The health of sexual minorities: Public health perspectives on lesbian, gay, bisexual and transgender populations*. New York: Springer.

Schaafsma, D. (2013). *Sexuality and intellectual disability: Implications for sex education*. Maastricht: Universitaire Pers Maastricht.

Schaafsma, D., Kok, G., Stoffelen, J. M. T., & Curfs, L. M. G. (2017). People with intellectual disabilities talk about sexuality: Implications for the development of sex education. *Sexuality and Disability, 35*(1), 21–38. http://dx.doi.org/10.1007/s11195-016-9466-4.

Schaafsma, D., Kok, G., Stoffelen, J. M. T., van Doorn, P., & Curfs, L. M. G. (2014). Identifying the important determinants of teaching sex education to people with intellectual disabilities: Cross-sectional survey among paid care staff. *Journal of Intellectual & Developmental Disability, 39*(2), 157–166. http://dx.doi.org/10.3109/13668250.2014.899566.

Schaafsma, D., Stoffelen, J. M. T., Kok, G., & Curfs, L. M. G. (2013). Exploring the development of existing sex education programs for people with intellectual disabilities: An intervention mapping approach. *Journal of Applied Research in Intellectual Disabilities, 26*, 157–166. http://dx.doi.org/10.1111/jar.12017.

Schalock, R., Luckasson, R., Bradley, V., Buntinx, W., Lachapelle, Y., Shogren, K. A., … Wehmeyer, M. L. (2012). *User's guide to accompany the 11th edition of intellectual disability: Definition, classification, and systems of supports. Applications for clinicians, educators, organizations providing supports, policymakers, family members and advocates, and health care professionals*. Washington: AAIDD.

Schalock, R. L., Borthwick-Duffy, S. A., Bradley, V. J., Buntinx, W. H. E., Coulter, D. L., Craig, E. M., ... Yeager, M. H. (2010). *Intellectual disability: Definition, classification, and systems of supports (11th ed. of AAIDD definition manual)*. Washington, DC US: American Association on Intellectual and Developmental Disabilities.

Scharlo, S., Ebbers, S., & Spijker, M. (2014). *SOS Snelle opvang bij seksueel misbruik van mensen met een verstandelijke beperking* [*SOS rapid care for sexual abuse of people with intellectual disabilities*]. Houten: Bohn, Stafleu, Van Loghum.

Sequeira, H., Howlin, P., & Hollins, S. (2003). Psychological disturbance associated with sexual abuse in people with learning disabilities: Case-control study. *The British Journal of Psychiatry, 183*, 451–456. http://dx.doi.org/10.1192/bjp.183.5.451.

Shakespeare, T. (2006). *Disability rights and wrongs*. Oxon: Routledge.

Siebelink, E. M., de Jong, M. D. T., Taal, E., & Roelvink, L. (2006). Sexuality and people with intellectual disabilities: Assessment of knowledge, attitudes, experiences, and needs. *Mental Retardation, 44*, 283–294. http://dx.doi.org/10.1352/0047-6765(2006)44[283:SAPWID]2.0.CO;2.

Stainton, T., & Clare, I. C. H. (2012). Human rights and intellectual disabilities: An emergent theoretical paradigm? *Journal of Intellectual Disability Research, 56*(11), 1011–1013. http://dx.doi.org/10.1111/Jir.12001.

Stoffelen, J., Kok, G., Hospers, H., & Curfs, L. M. G. (2013). Homosexuality among people with a mild intellectual disability: An explorative study on the lived experiences of homosexual people in The Netherlands with a mild intellectual disability. *Journal of Intellectual Disability Research, 57*, 257–267. http://dx.doi.org/10.1111/j.1365-2788.2011.01532.x.

Stoffelen, J. M. T., Schaafsma, D., Kok, G., & Curfs, L. M. G. (2017). *Women who love. An explorative study on the lived experiences of lesbian and bisexual women with a mild intellectual disability in The Netherlands*.

Streissguth, A. P., Bookstein, F. L., Barr, H. M., Sampson, P. D., O'Malley, K., & Kogan Young, J. (2004). Risk factors for adverse life outcomes in fetal alcohol syndrome and fetal alcohol effects. *Journal of Developmental & Behavioral Pediatrics, 25*(4), 228–238.

Swango-Wilson, A. (2008). Caregiver perception of sexual behaviours of individuals with intellectual disabilities. *Sexuality and Disability, 26*, 75–81. http://dx.doi.org/10.1007/s11195-008-9071-2.

Thompson, S. A. (2007). De/centering straight talk: Queerly informed inclusive pedagogy of gay and bisexual students with intellectual disabilities. *Journal of LGBT Youth, 5*, 37–56.

Thompson, S. A., Bryson, M., & de Castell, S. (2001). Prospects for identity formation for lesbian, gay, or bisexual persons with developmental disabilities. *International Journal of Disability, Development and Education, 48*, 53–65. http://dx.doi.org/10.1080/10349120120036305.

Van Berlo, W., de Haas, S., van Oosten, N., van Dijk, L., Brants, L., Tonnon, S., & Storms, O. (2011). *Beperkt weerbaar: Een onderzoek naar seksueel geweld bij mensen met een lichamelijk, zintuiglijk of een verstandelijke beperking* [*Sexual violence among individuals with a physical, sensory, or intellectual disability*]. Utrecht: van Berlo.

Van Doorn, P., van den Bogaard, K., & Embregts, P. (2014). Seks hoort ook bij mij. In P. Leusink, & M. Ramakers (red) (Eds.), *Handboek Seksuele gezondheid. Probleemgeoriënteerd denken en handelen [Sexual health handbook. Problem oriented thinking and acting]* (pp. 240–261). Assen: Koninklijke Van Gorcum.

Van Zenderen, K., & Hehenkamp, L. (2015). *SHVB-registratie 2011–2014* [*Registration of sex counseling to people with intellectual disability 20112014*]. Utrecht: Rutgers WPF.

Vanwesenbeeck, I. (2006). Seksuele diversiteit [Sexual diversity]. In L. Gijs, W. Gianotten, I. Vanwesenbeeck, & P. Weijenborg (red) (Eds.), *Seksuologie [sexology]*. Houten: Bohn Stafleu van Loghum.

Veltman, J. A., & Brunner, H. G. (2012). De novo mutations in human genetic disease. *Nature Reviews Genetics, 13*(8), 565–575.
Watson, S. L., Venema, T., Molloy, W., & Reich, M. (2002). Sexual rights and individuals who have a developmental disability. In D. M. Griffits, D. Richards, P. Fedoroff, & S. L. Watson (Eds.), *Ethical dilemmas: Sexuality and developmental disability* (pp. 19–53). New York: NADD Press.
Westheimer, R. K. (2005). The place of sexuality in our lives. In R. K. Westheimer, & S. Lopater (Eds.), *Human sexuality. A psychosocial perspective* (pp. 1–22). Baltimore & Philadelphia: Lippincott, Williams & Wilkins.
Wilkinson, V. J., Theodore, K., & Raczka, R. (2015). 'As normal as possible': Sexual identity development in people with intellectual disabilities transitioning to adulthood. *Sexuality and Disability, 33*(1), 93–105. http://dx.doi.org/10.1007/s11195-014-9356-6.
Wilson, N. (2009). *"Conditionally sexual": Constructing the sexual health needs of men and teenage boys with a moderate to profound intellectual disability*. Syndey: University of Sydney.
World Association for Sexual Health. (2014). *Declaration of sexual rights.*
World Health Organization. (2015). *Sexual health, human rights and the law.* Geneva: WHO. Retrieved from http://www.who.int/reproductivehealth/publications/sexual_health/sexual-health-human-rights-law/en/.
World Health Organization. (2016). *International statistical classification of diseases and related health problems 10th revision.* Geneva: World Health Organization.
Yool, L., Langdon, P. E., & Garner, K. (2003). The attitudes of medium-secure unit staff toward the sexuality of adults with learning disabilities. *Sexuality and Disability, 21*(2), 137–151. http://dx.doi.org/10.1023/A:1025499417787.
Young, R., Gore, N., & McCarthy, M. (2012). Staff attitudes towards sexuality in relation to gender of people with intellectual disability: A qualitative study. *Journal of Intellectual & Developmental Disability, 37*(4), 343–347.

FURTHER READING

World Health Organization. Sexual and reproductive health. Defining sexual health. Retrieved from http://www.who.int/reproductivehealth/topics/sexual_health/sh_definitions/en/.

FSC
www.fsc.org
MIX
Papier | Fördert
gute Waldnutzung
FSC® C083411

Kolibri 360 GmbH
Ferdinand-Jühlke-Straße 7
99095 Erfurt, Deutschland
produktsicherheit@kolibri360.de